DASH DIET
COOKBOOK

Recipes

Shrimp & Nectarine Salad

INGREDIENTS

1/3 cup orange juice
1 tablespoon minced fresh tarragon
1-1/2 teaspoons Dijon mustard
1-1/2 teaspoons honey
3 tablespoons cider vinegar
SALAD:
1/4 teaspoon salt
1/2 teaspoon lemon-pepper seasoning
1/2 cup finely chopped red onion
1 cup grape tomatoes, halved
1 cup fresh corn
1 pound uncooked shrimp (26-30 per pound), peeled and deveined
2 medium nectarines, cut into 1-inch pieces
4 teaspoons canola oil, divided
8 cups torn mixed salad greens

STEPS

1. In a bowl, whisk the vinegar, orange juice, honey, and mustard, until blended. Stir in tarragon.
2. In a skillet, heat 1 teaspoon oil over medium heat. Add corn; cook and stir for 2 minutes. Remove from pan.
3. Sprinkle shrimp with lemon pepper and salt. In the same skillet, heat the remaining oil over medium heat. Add shrimp; cook and stir for 4 minutes. Stir in corn.
4. In another bowl, combine the red onion, grape tomatoes, nectarines, salad green. Sprinkle with 1/3 cup dressing and toss to coat. Divide mixture among four plates. Garnish with shrimp mixture; drizzle with remaining dressing.
5. Serve immediately!

NUTRITION FACTS

Per Serving:
Calories: 252
Fat: 7 g
Saturated fat: 1 g
Carbohydrate: 27 g
Sodium: 448 mg
Cholesterol: 138 mg
Fiber: 5 g

Pork Chops with Tomato Curry

INGREDIENTS

1/2 teaspoon salt
1/2 teaspoon chili powder
1 small onion, finely chopped
2 tablespoons toasted slivered almonds
2 teaspoons curry powder
3 medium apples, thinly sliced
4 teaspoons butter, divided
4 teaspoons sugar
4 cups hot cooked brown rice
6 boneless pork loin chops
28 ounces whole tomatoes, undrained

STEPS

1. In a 6-qt. stockpot, heat 2 teaspoons butter over medium heat. Brown pork chops in batches. Remove from pan.
2. In the same pan, heat the remaining butter over medium heat. Add onion; cook and stir for 3 minutes. Stir in tomatoes, apples, curry powder, sugar, salt, and chili powder. Bring to a boil, stirring to break up tomatoes.
3. Return chops to pan. Reduce heat; simmer, uncovered, for 6 minutes. Turn chops; cook for about 6 minutes longer.
4. Serve with rice and, sprinkle with almonds.

NUTRITION FACTS

Per Serving:
Calories: 478
Fat: 14 g
Saturated fat: 5 g
Carbohydrates: 50 g
Sodium: 475 mg
Cholesterol: 89 mg
Fiber: 7 g

Sweet Oatmeal

INGREDIENTS

1/3 cup old-fashioned oats
1/2 cup assorted fresh fruit
1 tablespoon honey
2 tablespoons chopped walnuts, toasted
3 tablespoons fat-free milk
3 tablespoons reduced-fat plain yogurt

STEPS

1. In a container, combine oats, yogurt, milk, and honey.
2. Garnish with fruit and nuts.
3. Refrigerate overnight.

NUTRITION FACTS

Per Serving:
Calories: 345
Fat: 13 g
Saturated fat: 2 g
Carbohydrates: 53 g
Fiber: 5 g
Sodium: 53 mg
Cholesterol: 4 mg

Thai with Chicken and Pasta

INGREDIENTS

1 cup Thai peanut sauce
1 medium cucumber, halved lengthwise, seeded and sliced diagonally
2 teaspoons canola oil
2 cups julienned carrots
2 cups shredded cooked chicken
6 ounces uncooked whole wheat spaghetti
10 ounces fresh sugar snap peas, trimmed and cut diagonally into thin strips
Chopped fresh cilantro

STEPS

1. Cook spaghetti according to package directions; drain.
2. Meanwhile, in a skillet, heat oil over medium heat. Add carrots, and snap peas; stir-fry for 8 minutes. Add chicken, peanut sauce, and spaghetti; heat through, tossing to combine.
3. Transfer to a serving plate.
4. Garnish with cucumber and, cilantro. Serve!

NUTRITION FACTS

Per Serving:
Calories: 403
Fat: 15 g
Saturated fat: 3 g
Carbohydrates: 43 g
Fiber: 6 g
Sodium: 432 mg
Cholesterol: 42 mg

Chili-Lime Grilled Pineapple

INGREDIENTS

1 fresh pineapple
1 tablespoon lime juice
1 tablespoon olive oil
1 tablespoon honey
1-1/2 teaspoons chili powder
3 tablespoons brown sugar
Dash salt

STEPS

1. Peel pineapple, removing any eyes from fruit. Cut lengthwise into 6 wedges; remove the core.
2. In a bowl, mix the lime juice, olive oil, honey, chili powder, brown sugar, and salt, until blended. Brush pineapple with half of the glaze; reserve the remaining mixture for basting.
3. Grill pineapple, covered, over medium from heat for 4 minutes on each side, basting occasionally with reserved glaze.
4. Serve!

NUTRITION FACTS

Per Serving:
Calories: 97
Fat: 2 g
Saturated fat: 0 g
Carbohydrates: 20 g
Fiber: 1 g
Sodium: 35 mg
Cholesterol: 0 mg

Italian Sausage-Stuffed Zucchini

INGREDIENTS

3/4 cup shredded part-skim mozzarella cheese
1/4 teaspoon pepper
1/3 cup grated Parmesan cheese
1/3 cup minced fresh parsley
1 cup panko bread crumbs
1 pound Italian turkey sausage links, casings removed
2 medium tomatoes, seeded and chopped
2 tablespoons minced fresh oregano 2 tablespoons minced fresh basil
6 medium zucchini
Additional minced fresh parsley

NUTRITION FACTS

Per Serving:
Calories: 206
Fat: 9 g
Saturated fat: 3 g
Carbohydrates: 16 g
Fiber: 3 g
Sodium: 485 mg
Cholesterol: 39 mg

STEPS

1. Preheat oven to 375 degrees F. Cut each zucchini lengthwise in half. Scoop out pulp, leaving a 1/4-in. shell; chop pulp. Place zucchini shells in a large microwave-safe dish. In batches, microwave, covered, on high 3 minutes.
2. In a skillet, cook sausage and zucchini pulp over medium heat for about 9 minutes, breaking sausage into crumbles; drain. Stir in tomatoes, bread crumbs, Parmesan cheese, herbs, and pepper. Spoon into zucchini shells.
3. Place in 2 ungreased 13x9-in. baking dishes. Bake, covered, for 20 minutes. Sprinkle with mozzarella cheese. Bake, uncovered, for 7 minutes longer. Garnish with additional minced parsley.
4. Serve!

Spicy Almonds

INGREDIENTS

1/4 teaspoon cayenne pepper
1/2 teaspoon ground cinnamon
1/2 teaspoon ground cumin
1/2 teaspoon ground coriander
1 teaspoon paprika
1 large egg white, room temperature
1 tablespoon sugar
1-1/2 teaspoons kosher salt
2-1/2 cups unblanched almonds

STEPS

1. Preheat oven to 350 degrees F.
2. In a bowl, combine the salt, paprika, sugar, cinnamon, cumin, coriander, and cayenne pepper.
3. In another bowl, whisk egg white until foamy. Add almonds; toss to coat. Sprinkle with spice mixture; toss to coat.
4. Spread in a single layer in a greased baking pan.
5. Bake for about 25 minutes, stirring every 10 minutes. Spread on waxed paper to cool completely.
6. Store in an airtight container.

NUTRITION FACTS

Per Serving:
Calories: 230
Fat: 20 g
Saturated fat: 2 g
Carbohydrates: 9 g
Fiber: 4 g
Sodium: 293 mg
Cholesetrol: 0 mg

Lentil Salad

INGREDIENTS

1/4 cup minced fresh mint
1/2 cup rice vinegar
1/2 cup chopped soft sun-dried tomato halves
1 teaspoon dried basil
1 teaspoon dried oregano
1 medium cucumber, cubed
1 medium zucchini, cubed
1 small red onion, chopped
1 cup dried lentils, rinsed
2 cups water
2 cups sliced fresh mushrooms
2 teaspoons honey
3 tablespoons olive oil
4 cups fresh baby spinach, chopped
4 ounces crumbled feta cheese
4 bacon strips, cooked and crumbled

STEPS

1. Place lentils in a saucepan. Add water; bring to a boil. Reduce heat; simmer, covered, for 25 minutes. Drain and rinse in cold water.
2. Transfer to a bowl. Add onion, zucchini, mushrooms, cucumber, and tomatoes. In another bowl, whisk oil, vinegar, mint, honey, basil, and oregano.
3. Sprinkle over lentil mixture; toss to coat. Add spinach, cheese and, bacon; toss to combine.
4. Serve!

NUTRITION FACTS

Per Serving:
Calories: 225
Fat: 8 g
Saturated fat: 2 g
Carbohydrates: 29 g
Fiber: 5 g
Sodium: 400 mg
Cholesterol: 8 mg

Spiced Salmon

INGREDIENTS

1/4 teaspoon dill weed
1/2 teaspoon garlic powder
1/2 teaspoon ground mustard
1/2 teaspoon paprika
1/2 teaspoon pepper
1 salmon fillet
1 tablespoon soy sauce
1 tablespoon butter, melted
1 tablespoon olive oil
2 tablespoons packed brown sugar
Dash salt
Dash dried tarragon
Dash cayenne pepper

STEPS

1. Mix the dill weed, garlic powder, ground mustard, paprika, pepper, soy sauce, butter, olive oil, brown sugar, salt, tarragon, and cayenne pepper; brush over salmon.
2. Place salmon, skin side down, on an oiled grill rack. Grill, covered, over medium heat, for about 15 minutes.
3. Serve!

NUTRITION FACTS

Per Serving:
Calories: 256
Fat: 17 g
Saturated fat: 4 g
Carbohydrates: 5 g
Fiber: 0 g
Sodium: 330 mg
Cholesterol: 65 mg

Tomato and Green Bean Soup

INGREDIENTS

1/4 teaspoon pepper
1/4 cup minced fresh basil
1/2 teaspoon salt
1 cup chopped onion
1 cup chopped carrots
1 pound fresh green beans, cut into 1-inch pieces
1 garlic clove, minced
2 teaspoons butter
3 cups diced fresh tomatoes
6 cups vegetable broth

STEPS

1. In a saucepan, saute onion and carrots in butter for 6 minutes. Stir in the broth, beans, and garlic; bring to a boil. Reduce heat; cover and simmer for 25 minutes.
2. Stir in the tomatoes, basil, salt, and pepper. Cover and simmer 6 minutes longer.
3. Serve!

NUTRITION FACTS

Per Serving:
Calories: 58
Fat: 1 g
Saturated fat: 1 g
Carbohydrates: 10 g
Fiber: 3 g
Sodium: 535 mg
Cholesterol: 2 mg

Bean Hummus

INGREDIENTS

1/4 cup tahini
1/4 teaspoon salt
1/4 teaspoon crushed red pepper flakes
1-1/2 teaspoons ground cumin
2 garlic cloves, peeled
2 tablespoons minced fresh parsley
3 tablespoons lemon juice
15 ounces cannellini beans, rinsed and drained
Pita breads, cut into wedges
Assorted fresh vegetables

STEPS

1. Place garlic in a food processor; cover and process until minced. Add the lemon juice, beans, tahini, cumin, salt, and pepper flakes; cover and process until smooth.
2. Transfer to a bowl; stir in parsley. Refrigerate until serving.
3. Serve with pita wedges and assorted fresh vegetables.

NUTRITION FACTS

Per Serving:
Calories: 78
Fat: 4 g
Saturated fat: 1 g
Carbohydrates: 8 g
Sodium: 114 mg
Fiber: 2 g
Cholesterol: 0 mg

Sole with Pepper

INGREDIENTS

1/8 teaspoon cayenne pepper
1/4 teaspoon paprika
1/4 teaspoon lemon-pepper seasoning
1 medium tomato, chopped
2 tablespoons butter
2 cups sliced fresh mushrooms
2 garlic cloves, minced
2 green onions, thinly sliced
4 sole fillets

STEPS

1. In a skillet, heat butter over medium heat. Add mushrooms; cook and stir until tender. Add garlic; cook 1 minute longer.
2. Place fillets over mushrooms. Sprinkle with lemon pepper, paprika, and cayenne.
3. Cook, covered, over medium heat for 12 minutes.
4. Garnish with tomato and green onions.
5. Serve!

NUTRITION FACTS

Per Serving:
Calories: 174
Fat: 7 g
Saturated fat: 4 g
Carbohydrates: 4 g
Fiber: 1 g
Sodium: 166 mg
Cholesterol: 69 mg

Portobello Mushrooms Florentine

INGREDIENTS

1/8 teaspoon salt
1/8 teaspoon pepper
1/8 teaspoon garlic salt
1/4 cup crumbled feta cheese
1/2 teaspoon olive oil
1 small onion, chopped
1 cup fresh baby spinach
2 large portobello mushrooms, stems removed
2 large eggs
Minced fresh basil
Cooking spray

STEPS

1. Preheat oven to 450 degrees F. Sprinkle mushrooms with cooking spray; place in a baking pan, stem side up. Sprinkle with garlic salt and pepper. Bake, uncovered, for about 8 minutes.
2. Meanwhile, in a nonstick skillet, heat oil over medium heat; saute onion for 3 minutes. Stir in spinach until wilted.
3. Whisk together eggs and salt; add to skillet. Cook and stir until eggs are thickened; spoon onto mushrooms.
4. Garnish with cheese and, basil. Serve!

NUTRITION FACTS

Per Serving:
Calories: 126
Fat: 5 g
Saturated fat: 2 g
Carbohydrates: 10 g
Fiber: 3 g
Sodium: 472 mg
Cholesterol: 18 mg

Spinach-Stuffed Mushrooms

INGREDIENTS

1/8 teaspoon salt
1/2 cup water
1 tablespoon extra-virgin olive oil
8 large mushrooms
10 ounces frozen chopped spinach

STEPS

1. In a saucepan, bring 1/2 cup water to a boil. Add the spinach and salt. Cover, and cook according to package directions. Wash the mushrooms. Remove the stems, trim off the ends, then chop the stems.
2. Heat the olive oil in a skillet. Add the chopped mushroom stems. Sauté until golden, for 4 minutes. Remove from the pan. Add the mushroom caps to the skillet and sauté for 5 minutes. Remove the mushroom caps to a heatproof serving platter.
3. Drain the spinach. Stir in the sautéed chopped mushrooms.
4. Spoon the spinach mixture into the cups and serve immediately.

NUTRITION FACTS

Per Serving:
Calories: 33
Fat: 2 g
Carbohydrates: 3 g
Fiber: 2 g
Protein: 2 g
Sodium: 74 mg
Cholesterol: 0 mg

Shrimp Orzo with Feta

INGREDIENTS

1/4 teaspoon pepper
1/2 cup crumbled feta cheese
1-1/4 cups uncooked whole wheat orzo pasta
1-1/4 pounds uncooked shrimp (26-30 per pound), peeled and deveined
2 tablespoons olive oil
2 garlic cloves, minced
2 medium tomatoes, chopped
2 tablespoons lemon juice
2 tablespoons minced fresh cilantro

STEPS

1. Cook orzo according to package directions. Meanwhile, in a skillet, heat oil over medium heat. Add garlic; cook and stir for 1 minute. Add tomatoes and lemon juice.
2. Bring to a boil. Stir in shrimp. Reduce heat; simmer, uncovered, for about 5 minutes.
3. Drain orzo. Add orzo, cilantro, and pepper to shrimp mixture; heat through.
4. Garnish with feta cheese. Serve!

NUTRITION FACTS

Per Serving:
Calories: 406
Fat: 12 g
Saturated fat: 3 g
Carbohydrates: 40 g
Fiber: 9 g
Sodium: 307 mg
Cholesterol: 180 mg

Grilled Tomatoes

INGREDIENTS

2 large ripe red tomatoes, halved horizontally
Pinch salt
Pinch freshly ground black pepper

STEPS

1. Place the tomatoes on a grill, put sides facing up. Sprinkle with salt and pepper.
2. Broil for 10 minutes.
3. Serve!

NUTRITION FACTS

Per Serving:
Calories: 38
Fat: 1 g
Carbohydrates: 8 g
Fiber: 2 g
Protein: 2 g
Sodium: 16 mg
Cholesterol: 0 mg

Penne with Beef and Blue Cheese

INGREDIENTS

1/4 teaspoon salt
1/4 teaspoon pepper
1/4 cup chopped walnuts
1/4 cup crumbled Gorgonzola cheese
1/3 cup prepared pesto
2 cups uncooked whole wheat penne pasta
2 beef tenderloin steaks
2 cups grape tomatoes, halved
6 cups fresh baby spinach, coarsely chopped

STEPS

1. Cook pasta according to package directions.
2. Meanwhile, drizzle steaks with salt and pepper. Grill steaks, covered, over medium heat for 7 minutes on each side.
3. Drain pasta; transfer to a bowl. Add tomatoes, spinach, pesto, and walnuts; toss to coat. Cut steak into thin slices.
4. Serve pasta mixture with beef.
5. Garnish with blue cheese.

NUTRITION FACTS

Per Serving:
Calories: 532
Fat: 22 g
Saturated fat: 6 g
Carbohydrates: 49 g
Fiber: 9 g
Sodium: 434 mg
Cholesterol: 50 mg

Citrus Pork Roast

INGREDIENTS

1/2 teaspoon salt
1/2 teaspoon pepper
1/2 teaspoon ground ginger
1 boneless pork sirloin roast
1 teaspoon dried oregano
1 tablespoon sugar
1 tablespoon white grapefruit juice
1 tablespoon steak sauce
1 tablespoon reduced-sodium soy sauce
1 teaspoon grated orange zest
1 cup plus 3 tablespoons orange juice, divided
2 medium onions, cut into thin wedges
3 tablespoons cornstarch
Hot cooked egg noodles
Minced fresh oregano

NUTRITION FACTS

Per Serving:
Calories: 289
Fat: 10 g
Saturated fat: 4 g
Carbohydrates: 13 g
Fiber: 1 g
Sodium: 326 mg
Cholesterol: 102 mg

STEPS

1. Cut roast in half. In a bowl, combine the ginger, oregano, and pepper; rub over pork. In a nonstick skillet coated with cooking spray, brown roast on all sides. Transfer to a 4-qt. slow cooker; add onions.
2. In another bowl, combine 1 cup orange juice, grapefruit juice, steak sauce, sugar, and soy sauce; pour over top. Cover and cook on low for about 4 hours. Remove meat and onions to a serving platter; keep warm.
3. Skim fat from cooking juices; transfer to a small saucepan. Add orange zest and salt. Bring to a boil. Combine cornstarch and the remaining orange juice until smooth. Gradually stir into the pan. Bring to a boil; cook and stir for 3 minutes.
4. Serve with pork and noodles. Garnish with fresh oregano. Serve!

Asparagus with Horseradish Dip

INGREDIENTS

1/4 cup grated Parmesan cheese
1/2 teaspoon Worcestershire sauce
1 cup reduced-fat mayonnaise
1 tablespoon prepared horseradish
2 pounds fresh asparagus spears, trimmed

STEPS

1. Place asparagus in a steamer basket; place in a saucepan over 1 in. of water.
2. Bring to a boil; cover and steam until crisp-tender, for 4 minutes. Drain and immediately place in ice water. Drain and pat dry.
3. In a bowl, combine the Parmesan cheese, mayonnaise, Worcestershire sauce, and horseradish, mix.
4. Serve with asparagus.

NUTRITION FACTS

Per Serving:
Calories: 136
Fat: 10 g
Saturated fat: 2 g
Carbohydrates: 6 g
Fiber: 0 g
Sodium: 290 mg
Cholesterol: 12 mg

Grilled Tilapia with Pineapple Sauce

INGREDIENTS

1/8 teaspoon plus 1/4 teaspoon salt, divided
1/8 teaspoon pepper
1/4 cup finely chopped green pepper
1/4 cup minced fresh cilantro
1 tablespoon canola oil
2 cups cubed fresh pineapple
2 green onions, chopped
4 teaspoons plus 2 tablespoons lime juice, divided
8 tilapia fillets
Dash cayenne pepper

STEPS

1. For salsa, in a bowl, combine green onions, pineapple, green pepper, cilantro, 4 teaspoons lime juice, 1/8 teaspoon salt, and cayenne. Refrigerate until serving.
2. Mix oil and remaining lime juice; drizzle over fillets. Sprinkle with pepper and remaining salt.
3. Grill fish, covered, on an oiled rack over medium heat, for 3 minutes on each side.
4. Serve with salsa!

NUTRITION FACTS

Per Serving:
Calories: 131
Fat: 3 g
Saturated fat: 1 g
Carbohydrates: 6 g
Fiber: 1 g
Sodium: 152 mg
Cholesterol: 55 mg

California-Style Quinoa

INGREDIENTS

3/4 cup canned garbanzo beans, rinsed and drained
1/4 cup finely chopped Greek olives
1/4 teaspoon pepper
1/2 cup crumbled feta cheese
1 tablespoon olive oil
1 cup quinoa, rinsed and well drained
1 medium zucchini, chopped
1 medium tomato, finely chopped
2 garlic cloves, minced
2 cups water
2 tablespoons minced fresh basil

STEPS

1. In a saucepan, heat oil over medium heat. Add quinoa and garlic; cook and stir for 3 minutes. Stir in zucchini and water; bring to a boil.
2. Reduce heat; simmer, covered, for about 15 minutes. Stir in the garbanzo beans, Greek olives, feta cheese, 1 tablespoon fresh basil, and tomato; heat through.
3. Garnish with remaining fresh basil. Serve!

NUTRITION FACTS

Per Serving:
Calories: 310
Fat: 11 g
Saturated fat: 3 g
Carbohydrates: 42 g
Fiber: 6 g
Sodium: 353 mg
Cholesterol: 8 mg

Peppered Tuna Kabobs

INGREDIENTS

1/2 cup frozen corn, thawed
1 teaspoon coarsely ground pepper
1 jalapeno pepper, seeded and chopped
1 pound tuna steaks, cut into 1-inch cubes
1 medium mango, peeled and cut into 1-inch cubes
2 tablespoons coarsely chopped fresh parsley
2 tablespoons lime juice
2 large sweet red peppers, cut into 2x1-inch pieces
4 green onions, chopped

STEPS

1. For salsa, in a bowl, combine the lemon juice, corn, green onions, parsley, and jalapeno pepper; set aside.
2. Drizzle tuna with pepper. On four soaked wooden skewers, alternately thread red peppers, tuna, and mango.
3. Place skewers on greased grill rack. Cook, covered, over medium heat, turning occasionally, for 12 minutes.
4. Serve with salsa!

NUTRITION FACTS

Per Serving:
Calories: 205
Fat: 2 g
Saturated fat: 0 g
Carbohydrates: 20 g
Fiber: 4 g
Sodium: 50 mg
Cholesterol: 51 mg

Poached Salmon with Spinach Salad

INGREDIENTS

1/8 teaspoon freshly ground black pepper
1/4 teaspoon salt
1/2 pound cleaned fresh spinach
1/2 cup chopped yellow onion
1 tablespoon coarsely chopped flat-leaf parsley
2 tablespoons extra-virgin olive oil
3 fresh tomatoes, peeled, seeded and cut into 1/2" pieces
Poached salmon

STEPS

1. In a skillet, heat 1 tablespoon of the oil over medium heat. When hot, sauté the spinach for 2 minutes. Add in the salt and pepper and divide the spinach among 4 plates.
2. Heat the remaining tablespoon of oil in the skillet. Sauté the onion and tomatoes over medium heat, about 6 minutes.
3. Arrange the salmon on the spinach and top with the tomatoes and onion.
4. Garnish with parsley.
5. Serve!

NUTRITION FACTS

Per Serving:
Calories: 98
Fat: 7 g
Carbohydrates: 9 g
Fiber: 2 g
Protein: 2 g
Sodium: 162 mg
Cholesterol: 0 mg

Cherry-Chicken Lettuce Wraps

INGREDIENTS

1/4 teaspoon salt
1/4 teaspoon pepper
1/3 cup coarsely chopped almonds
3/4 pound boneless skinless chicken breasts, cut into 3/4-inch cubes
1 tablespoon honey
1 teaspoon ground ginger
1-1/2 cups shredded carrots
1-1/4 cups coarsely chopped pitted fresh sweet cherries
2 teaspoons olive oil
2 tablespoons rice vinegar
2 tablespoons reduced-sodium teriyaki sauce
4 green onions, chopped
8 Bibb lettuce leaves

STEPS

1. Sprinkle chicken with ginger, salt, and pepper. In a nonstick skillet, heat oil over medium heat. Add chicken; cook and stir for 5 minutes.
2. Remove from heat. Stir in carrots, green onions, cherries, and almonds.
3. In a bowl, mix the teriyaki sauce, vinegar, and honey; stir into the chicken mixture.
4. Divide among lettuce leaves; fold lettuce over filling.
5. Serve!

NUTRITION FACTS

Per Serving:
Calories: 257
Fat: 10 g
Saturated fat: 1 g
Carbohydrates: 22 g
Fiber: 4 g
Sodium: 381 mg
Cholesterol: 47 mg

Mango Rice Pudding

INGREDIENTS

1/4 teaspoon salt
1/2 teaspoon ground cinnamon
1 cup uncooked long grain brown rice
1 medium ripe mango
1 teaspoon vanilla extract
1 cup vanilla soy milk
2 cups water
2 tablespoons sugar
Chopped peeled mango

STEPS

1. In a saucepan, bring water and salt to a boil; stir in rice. Reduce heat; simmer, covered, for about 30 minutes.
2. Meanwhile, peel, seed, and slice mango. Mash mango with a potato masher.
3. Stir milk, sugar, cinnamon, and mashed mango into the rice. Cook, uncovered, on low for 15 minutes longer or until liquid is almost absorbed, stirring occasionally.
4. Remove from heat; stir in vanilla.
5. Garnish with chopped mango.
6. Serve!

NUTRITION FACTS

Per Serving:
Calories: 275
Fat: 3 g
Saturated fat: 0 g
Carbohydrates: 58 g
Fiber: 3 g
Sodium: 176 mg
Cholesterol: 0 mg

Asparagus Omelet Tortilla

INGREDIENTS

1/8 teaspoon pepper
1 teaspoon butter
1 green onion, chopped
1 whole wheat tortilla (8 inches), warmed
1 large egg
1 tablespoon fat-free milk
2 teaspoons grated Parmesan cheese
2 large egg whites
4 fresh asparagus spears, trimmed and sliced

STEPS

1. In a bowl, whisk the egg, egg whites, fat-free milk, Parmesan cheese, and pepper until blended. Place a nonstick skillet coated with cooking spray over medium heat; add asparagus. Cook and stir for 4 minutes. Remove from pan.
2. In the same skillet, heat butter over medium heat. Pour in egg mixture. The mixture should set immediately at the edges. As eggs set, push cooked portions toward the center, letting uncooked eggs flow underneath. When eggs are thickened and no liquid egg remains, spoon green onion and asparagus on one side.
3. Fold omelet in half; serve in a tortilla.

NUTRITION FACTS

Per Serving:
Calories: 319
Fat: 13 g
Saturated fat: 5 g
Carbohydrates: 28 g
Fiber: 3 g
Sodium: 444 mg
Cholesterol: 225 mg

Black Bean & White Cheddar Frittata

INGREDIENTS

1/4 teaspoon salt
1/4 teaspoon pepper
1/4 cup salsa
1/3 cup finely chopped green pepper
1/3 cup finely chopped sweet red pepper
1/2 cup shredded white cheddar cheese
1 cup canned black beans, rinsed and drained
1 tablespoon minced fresh parsley
1 tablespoon olive oil
2 garlic cloves, minced
3 green onions, finely chopped
3 large egg whites
6 large eggs
Minced fresh cilantro

STEPS

1. Preheat broiler. In a bowl, whisk the eggs, withes eggs, salsa, parsley, salt, and pepper, until blended.
2. In a skillet, heat oil over medium heat. Add peppers and green onions; cook and stir for 5 minutes. Add garlic; cook 1 minute longer. Stir in beans. Reduce heat to medium; stir in egg mixture. Cook, uncovered, for 6 minutes. Sprinkle with cheese.
3. Broil 3-4 in. from heat for 4 minutes.
4. Let stand 5 minutes. Cut into wedges.
5. Serve with fresh cilantro.

NUTRITION FACTS

Per Serving:
Calories: 183
Fat: 10 g
Saturated fat: 4 g
Carbohydrates: 9 g
Fiber: 2 g
Sodium: 378 mg
Cholesterol: 196 mg

Cobb Salad

INGREDIENTS

3/4 cup Asian toasted sesame salad dressing
1/4 cup fresh cilantro leaves
1/2 cup unsalted peanuts
1 bunch romaine, torn
1 medium ripe avocado, peeled and thinly sliced
1 medium carrot, shredded
1 medium sweet red pepper, julienned
1 cup fresh snow peas, halved
2 cups shredded rotisserie chicken
2 tablespoons creamy peanut butter
3 hard-boiled large eggs, coarsely chopped

STEPS

1. Place romaine on a large serving platter. Arrange chicken, vegetables, avocado, eggs, and peanuts over romaine; sprinkle with cilantro.
2. In a bowl, whisk salad dressing and peanut butter until smooth.
3. Serve with salad!

NUTRITION FACTS

Per Serving:
Calories: 382
Fat: 25 g
Saturated fat: 5 g
Carbohydrates: 18 g
Fiber: 5 g
Sodium: 472 mg
Cholesterol: 135 mg

Turkey and Vegetable Barley Soup

INGREDIENTS

2/3 cup quick-cooking barley
1/2 teaspoon pepper
1 medium onion, chopped
1 tablespoon canola oil
2 cups cubed cooked turkey breast
2 cups fresh baby spinach
5 medium carrots, chopped
6 cups reduced-sodium chicken broth

STEPS

1. In a saucepan, heat oil over medium heat. Add onion and carrots; cook and stir for 6 minutes.
2. Stir in barley and broth; bring to a boil. Reduce heat; simmer, covered, for about 16 minutes. Stir in turkey, spinach, and pepper; heat through.
3. Serve!

NUTRITION FACTS

Per Serving:
Calories: 208
Fat: 4 g
Saturated fat: 1 g
Carbohydrates: 23 g
Fiber: 6 g
Sodium: 662 mg
Cholesterol: 37 mg

Light & Creamy Chocolate Pudding

INGREDIENTS

1/8 teaspoon salt
1 teaspoon vanilla extract
2 tablespoons sugar
2 tablespoons baking cocoa
2 cups chocolate soy milk
3 tablespoons cornstarch

STEPS

1. In a saucepan, mix cornstarch, cocoa, sugar, and salt. Whisk in milk. Cook and stir over medium heat until thickened and bubbly. Reduce heat to low; cook and stir 2 minutes longer.
2. Remove from heat. Stir in vanilla. Cool 20 minutes, stirring occasionally.
3. Transfer to dessert dishes. Refrigerate, covered, for about 40 minutes.
4. Serve!

NUTRITION FACTS

Per Serving:
Calories: 127
Fat: 2 g
Saturated fat: 0 g
Carbohydrates: 25 g
Fiber: 1 g
Sodium: 112 mg
Cholesterol: 0 mg

Oriental Cabbage Salad

INGREDIENTS

1/2 small head green cabbage
2 tablespoons dark sesame oil
2 tablespoons rice wine vinegar
2 tablespoons sesame seeds, toasted
3 scallions, chopped

STEPS

1. Combine the scallions, cabbage, oil, and vinegar. Toss well and chill until ready to serve.
2. Add the sesame seeds and toss again before serving.

NUTRITION FACTS

Per Serving:
Calories: 103
Fat: 9 g
Carbohydrates: 5 g
Fiber: 2 g
Protein: 2 g
Sodium: 15 mg
Cholesterol: 0 mg

Grilled Steak Salad

INGREDIENTS

1/4 teaspoon salt
1/4 teaspoon ground cumin
1/4 teaspoon pepper
1 large sweet onion, cut into 1/2-inch rings
1 tablespoon olive oil
1 beef top sirloin steak
2 large ears sweet corn, husks removed
2 cups uncooked multigrain bow tie pasta
2 large tomatoes
3 poblano peppers, halved and seeded
DRESSING:
1/4 cup lime juice
1/4 teaspoon salt
1/4 teaspoon ground cumin
1/4 teaspoon pepper
1/3 cup chopped fresh cilantro
1 tablespoon olive oil

NUTRITION FACTS

Per Serving:
Calories: 546
Fat: 13 g
Saturated fat: 3 g
Carbohydrates: 58 g
Fiber: 8 g
Sodium: 378 mg
Cholesterol: 34 mg

STEPS

1. Rub steak with salt, cumin, and pepper. Brush poblano peppers, corn, and onion with oil. Grill steak, covered, over medium heat for about 8 minutes on each side. Grill vegetables, covered, for 10 minutes, turning occasionally.
2. Cook pasta according to package directions. Meanwhile, cut corn from the cob; coarsely chop onion, peppers, and tomatoes. Transfer vegetables to a large bowl. In another bowl, whisk oil, lime juice, cumin, salt, and pepper until blended; stir in cilantro.
3. Drain pasta; add to vegetable mixture. Sprinkle with the dressing; toss to coat. Cut steak into thin slices; add to salad.
4. Serve!

Grapefruit, Lime & Yogurt Parfait

INGREDIENTS

2 teaspoons grated lime zest
2 tablespoons lime juice
3 tablespoons honey
4 large red grapefruit
4 cups reduced-fat plain yogurt
Torn fresh mint leaves

STEPS

1. Cut a thin slice from the top and bottom of each grapefruit; stand fruit upright on a cutting board. With a knife, cut off the peel and outer membrane from the grapefruit. Cut along the membrane of each segment to remove the fruit.
2. In a bowl, mix yogurt, lime zest, and juice. Layer half of the grapefruit and half of the yogurt mixture into 6 parfait glasses. Repeat layers. Sprinkle with honey.
3. Garnish with mint. Serve!

NUTRITION FACTS

Per Serving:
Calories: 207
Fat: 3 g
Saturated fat: 2 g
Carbohydrates: 39 g
Fiber: 3 g
Sodium: 115 mg
Cholesterol: 10 mg

Cabbage Roll

INGREDIENTS

1/2 teaspoon pepper
1 pound extra-lean ground beef (95% lean)
1 tablespoon brown sugar
1 teaspoon dried oregano
1 teaspoon dried thyme
1 small head cabbage, thinly sliced
1 medium green pepper, cut into thin strips
1 large onion, chopped
2 tablespoons cider vinegar
4 cups hot cooked brown rice
8 ounces tomato sauce
28 ounces whole plum tomatoes, undrained

STEPS

1. Drain tomatoes, reserving liquid; coarsely chop tomatoes. In a nonstick skillet, cook the onion and beef over medium heat for 9 minutes, breaking up beef into crumbles. Stir in tomato sauce, vinegar, brown sugar, seasonings, chopped tomatoes, and reserved liquid.
2. Add cabbage and pepper; cook, covered, 6 minutes, stirring occasionally. Cook, uncovered, for 8 minutes.
3. Serve with rice.

NUTRITION FACTS

Per Serving:
Calories: 332
Fat: 5 g
Saturated fat: 2 g
Carbohydrates: 50 g
Fiber: 9 g
Sodium: 439 mg
Cholesterol: 43 mg

Layered Hummus Dip

INGREDIENTS

1/4 cup finely chopped red onion
1/2 cup Greek olives, chopped
1 large English cucumber, chopped
1 cup crumbled feta cheese
2 medium tomatoes, seeded and chopped
10 ounces hummus
Baked pita chips

STEPS

1. Spread hummus into a shallow 10-in. round dish. Layer with onion, tomatoes, olives, cucumber, and cheese. Refrigerate until serving.
2. Serve with pita chips.

NUTRITION FACTS

Per Serving:
Calories: 88
Fat: 5 g
Saturated fat: 2 g
Carbohydrates: 6 g
Fiber: 2 g
Sodium: 275 mg
Cholesterol: 5 mg

Warm Rice & Pintos Salad

INGREDIENTS

1/4 cup finely shredded cheddar cheese
1/4 cup chopped fresh cilantro
1/2 cup salsa
1 bunch romaine, quartered lengthwise through the core
1 tablespoon olive oil
1 cup frozen corn
1 small onion, chopped
1-1/2 teaspoons chili powder
1-1/2 teaspoons ground cumin
2 garlic cloves, minced
4 ounces chopped green chilies
8.8 ounces ready-to-serve brown rice
15 ounces pinto beans, rinsed and drained

STEPS

1. In a skillet, heat oil over medium heat. Add onion and corn; cook and stir for 6 minutes. Stir in garlic, chili powder, and cumin; cook and stir 1 minute longer.
2. Add beans, rice, green chilies, salsa, and cilantro; heat through, stirring occasionally.
3. Garnish with cheese.
4. Serve over romaine wedges.

NUTRITION FACTS

Per Serving:
Calories: 331
Fat: 8 g
Saturated fat: 2 g
Carbohydrates: 50 g
Fiber: 9 g
Sodium: 465 mg
Cholesterol: 7 mg

Crunchy Green Bean

INGREDIENTS

1/4 cup gorgonzola, crumbled
1/2 cup plain unsalted tortilla chips, crushed
1/2 cup panko breadcrumbs
2 tablespoons hot sauce
2 tablespoons butter, unsalted, melted
2 tablespoons green onions, chopped
12 oz of Fresh String green beans

STEPS

1. Preheat oven to 350 degrees F.
2. Chop green beans to ~2" pieces, steam for 6 minutes in a microwave-safe plate, damp moist paper towel.
3. Mix cut string green beans with the hot sauce. Pour mixture into a casserole dish.
4. Mix gorgonzola, tortilla chips, bread crumbs, butter, and green onions, in a bowl. Sprinkle mixture evenly over string green beans and bake green bean casserole uncovered in the oven for 20 minutes.
5. Serve!

NUTRITION FACTS

Per Serving:

Calories: 122
Fat: 6 g
Carbohydrates: 11 g
Fiber: 2.4 g
Protein: 4 g
Sodium: 221 mg

Delicious Hot Crab Dip

INGREDIENTS

1/4 teaspoon pepper
1/4 cup sour cream
1/4 cup mayonnaise
1/2 teaspoon salt
1/2 teaspoon paprika
1 cup cheddar cheese grated
1 teaspoon garlic powder
1 Tablespoon Worcestershire Sauce
1 Tablespoon lemon juice
1 pound lump crab meat canned
8 ounce cream cheese softened

STEPS

1. Preheat your oven to 375 degrees F.
2. In a mixing bowl, combine cream cheese, mayonnaise, sour cream, cheddar cheese, paprika, garlic powder, lemon juice, Worcestershire sauce, salt, and pepper. Stir together until combined and fold in lump crab meat.
3. Spread in a casserole dish and bake for 20 minutes.
4. Serve with tortilla chips!

NUTRITION FACTS

Per Serving:
Calories: 178
Fat: 7 g
Carbohydrates: 2 g
Fiber: 1 g
Protein: 11 g
Sodium: 580 mg
Cholesterol: 51 mg

Vegetable and Beef Soup

INGREDIENTS

1/4 teaspoon salt
1/4 teaspoon pepper
1/4 cup tomato paste
1/2 teaspoon dried oregano
1/2 cup fresh cut green beans
1 medium zucchini, coarsely chopped
1 medium red potato, finely chopped
1 teaspoon dried basil
1 medium onion, chopped
1-1/2 pounds lean ground beef (90% lean)
1-1/2 cups shredded cabbage
2 garlic cloves, minced
2 celery ribs, chopped
10 ounces julienned carrots
14-1/2 ounces diced tomatoes, undrained
14-1/2 ounces each reduced-sodium beef broth
Grated Parmesan cheese

STEPS

1. In a 6-qt. stockpot, cook beef, onion, and garlic over medium heat for 9 minutes, breaking up beef into crumbles; drain.
2. Add carrots and celery; cook and stir for 7 minutes. Stir in tomato paste; cook 1 minute longer.
3. Add potato, tomatoes, green beans, cabbage, zucchini, seasonings, and broth; bring to a boil. Reduce heat; simmer, covered, for 50 minutes.
4. Garnish each serving with cheese.
5. Serve!

NUTRITION FACTS

Per Serving:
Calories: 207
Fat: 7 g
Saturated fat: 3 g
Carbohydrates: 14 g
Fiber: 3 g
Sodium: 621 mg
Cholesterol: 57 mg

Raspberry Peach Puff Pancake

INGREDIENTS

1/8 teaspoon salt
1/4 cup vanilla yogurt
1/2 cup fat-free milk
1/2 cup all-purpose flour
1/2 teaspoon sugar
1/2 cup fresh raspberries
1 tablespoon butter
2 medium peaches, peeled and sliced
3 large eggs, room temperature, lightly beaten

STEPS

1. Preheat oven to 400 degrees F. In a bowl, toss peaches with sugar; gently stir in raspberries.
2. Place butter in a 9-in. pie plate; heat in oven until butter is melted, for about 3 minutes. Meanwhile, in a bowl, whisk milk, eggs, and salt until blended; gradually whisk in flour. Remove pie plate from oven; tilt carefully to coat bottom and sides with butter. Immediately pour in the egg mixture.
3. Bake until pancake is puffed and browned, for 22 minutes. Remove from oven.
4. Serve immediately with fruit and yogurt.

NUTRITION FACTS

Per Serving:
Calories: 199
Fat: 7 g
Saturated fat: 3 g
Carbohydrates: 25 g
Fiber: 3 g
Sodium: 173 mg
Cholesterol: 149 mg

Turkey and Basil Burgers

INGREDIENTS

1/8 teaspoon pepper
1/4 teaspoon garlic salt
1/4 cup chopped fresh basil
1 garlic clove, minced
1 pound lean ground turkey
2 tablespoons quick-cooking oats
3 tablespoons mesquite smoke-flavored barbecue sauce
4 whole-wheat hamburger buns, split
Red onion slices
Sliced tomato
Fresh basil leaves
Barbecue sauce

STEPS

1. In a bowl, combine oats, garlic salt, basil, barbecue sauce, garlic, and pepper. Add turkey; mix lightly. Shape into four 1/2-in.-thick patties.
2. On a lightly greased grill rack, grill burgers, covered, over medium heat for 7 minutes on each side. Grill buns over medium heat, cut side down, for about 60 seconds.
3. Serve burgers on buns with red onions, tomato, fresh basil, and barbecue sauce.

NUTRITION FACTS

Per Serving:
Calories: 315
Fat: 11 g
Saturated fat: 3 g
Carbohydrates: 29 g
Fiber: 4g
Sodium: 482 mg
Cholesterol: 78 mg

Strawberry-Blue Cheese Steak Salad

INGREDIENTS

1/4 teaspoon pepper
1/2 teaspoon salt
1 beef top sirloin steak (3/4 inch thick and 1 pound)
2 teaspoons olive oil
2 tablespoons lime juice
SALAD:
1/4 cup thinly sliced red onion
1/4 cup crumbled blue cheese
1/4 cup chopped walnuts, toasted
1 bunch romaine, torn
2 cups fresh strawberries, halved
Reduced-fat balsamic vinaigrette

STEPS

1. Season steak with salt and pepper. In a skillet, heat oil over medium heat. Add steak; cook for 7 minutes on each side.
2. Remove from pan; let stand 5 minutes. Cut steak into bite-sized strips; toss with lime juice.
3. On a platter, combine romaine, strawberries, and onion; top with steak.
4. Garnish with cheese and walnuts.
5. Serve with vinaigrette.

NUTRITION FACTS

Per Serving:
Calories: 289
Fat: 15 g
Saturated fat: 4 g
Carbohydrates: 12 g
Fiber: 4 g
Sodium: 452 mg
Cholesterol: 52 mg

Quinoa and Veggie Sauce

INGREDIENTS

3/4 cup peeled, seeded and finely chopped cucumber
3/4 cup finely chopped zucchini
2/3 cup quinoa, rinsed
1/4 cup finely chopped red onion
1/4 cup minced fresh cilantro
1/2 teaspoon cayenne pepper
1-1/2 teaspoons ground cumin
1-1/2 teaspoons paprika
1-2/3 cups water, divided
2 medium ripe avocados, peeled and coarsely chopped
2 tablespoons plus 3/4 cup sour cream, divided
3 plum tomatoes, chopped
5 tablespoons lime juice, divided
15 ounces black beans, rinsed and drained
Cucumber slices
Salt and pepper to taste

STEPS

1. Pulse beans, paprika, cumin, cayenne, and 1/3 cup water in a food processor until smooth. Add salt and pepper to taste.
2. In a saucepan, cook quinoa with the remaining 1-1/3 cups water according to package directions. Fluff with fork; sprinkle with 2 tablespoons lime juice. Set aside.
3. Meanwhile, mash together 2 tablespoons sour cream, avocados, cilantro, and remaining lime juice.
4. In a 2-1/2-qt. dish, layer bean mixture, quinoa, avocado mixture, remaining sour cream, tomatoes, zucchini, chopped cucumber, and onion.
5. Serve immediately with cucumber slices for dipping.

NUTRITION FACTS

Per Serving:
Calories: 65
Fat: 3 g
Saturated fat: 1 g
Carbohydrates: 8 g
Fiber: 2 g
Sodium: 54 mg
Cholesterol: 4 mg

Roasted Sweet Potato & Chickpea Pitas

INGREDIENTS

1/4 cup minced fresh cilantro
1/2 teaspoon salt, divided
1 cup plain Greek yogurt
1 tablespoon lemon juice
1 medium red onion, chopped
1 teaspoon ground cumin
2 medium sweet potatoes, peeled and cubed
2 teaspoons garam masala
2 garlic cloves, minced
2 cups arugula or baby spinach
3 tablespoons canola oil, divided
12 whole wheat pita pocket halves, warmed
15 ounces each chickpeas, rinsed and drained

STEPS

1. Preheat oven to 425 degrees F. Place potatoes in a microwave-safe bowl; microwave, covered, on high 5 minutes. Stir in chickpeas and onion; toss with 2 tablespoons oil, garam masala, and 1/4 teaspoon salt.
2. Spread into a pan. Roast, for about 15 minutes. Cool slightly.
3. Place garlic and remaining oil in another microwave-safe bowl; microwave on high, for 1 minute. Stir in lemon juice, yogurt, cumin, and remaining salt.
4. Toss potato mixture with arugula.
5. Spoon into pitas; garnish with sauce and cilantro. Serve!

NUTRITION FACTS

Per Serving:
Calories: 462
Fat: 15 g
Saturated fat: 3 g
Carbohydrates: 72 g
Fiber: 12 g
Sodium: 662 mg
Cholesterol: 10 mg

Chickpeas with Spinach & Bacon

INGREDIENTS

1/2 bag baby leaf spinach
1 rasher lean back bacon
1 thinly sliced garlic clove
1 tbsp wine vinegar
3 tbsp canned chickpeas, drained and washed
Salt and black pepper

STEPS

1. Cut the bacon rasher into strips and cook in a hot non-stick pan with the garlic clove. Add the wine vinegar, chickpeas, and spinach, stirring until wilted.
2. Season with salt and pepper.
3. Serve!

NUTRITION FACTS

Per Serving:
Calories: 97
Fat: 3 g
Carbohydrates: 9 g
Fiber: 2 g
Protein: 9 g
Sugars: 0 g
Sodium: 1.54 g

Brunch Banana Splits

INGREDIENTS

1/2 cup granola without raisins
1 cup fresh raspberries
2 cups fat-free vanilla Greek yogurt
2 small peaches, sliced
2 tablespoons sliced almonds, toasted
2 tablespoons sunflower kernels
2 tablespoons honey
4 small bananas, peeled and halved lengthwise

STEPS

1. Divide bananas among four shallow dishes.
2. Garnish with granola, raspberries, Greek yogurt, peaches, almonds, sunflower kernels, and honey.
3. Serve!

NUTRITION FACTS

Per Serving:
Calories: 340
Fat: 6 g
Saturated fat: 1 g
Carbohydrates: 61 g
Fiber: 9 g
Sodium: 88 mg
Cholesterol: 0 mg

Peach Tart

INGREDIENTS

1/4 teaspoon ground nutmeg
1/4 cup butter, softened
1 cup all-purpose flour
3 tablespoons sugar
FILLING:
1/8 teaspoon almond extract
1/4 teaspoon ground cinnamon
1/4 cup sliced almonds
1/3 cup sugar
2 pounds peaches, peeled and sliced
2 tablespoons all-purpose flour
Whipped cream

STEPS

1. Preheat oven to 375 degrees F. Cream butter, sugar, and nutmeg mix until light and fluffy, for 7 minutes. Beat in flour until blended. Press firmly onto the bottom and up sides of an ungreased 9-in. fluted tart pan with removable bottom.
2. Place on a baking sheet. Bake on the middle oven rack, for 12 minutes. Cool on a wire rack.
3. In a bowl, toss peaches with flour, sugar, cinnamon, and extract; add to crust. Sprinkle with almonds.
4. Bake tart on a lower oven rack, for about 45 minutes. Cool on a wire rack.
5. Garnish with whipped cream. Serve!

NUTRITION FACTS

Per Serving:
Calories: 222
Fat: 8 g
Saturated fat: 4 g
Carbohydrates: 36 g
Fiber: 3 g
Sodium: 46 mg
Cholesterol: 15 mg

Asparagus Soup

INGREDIENTS

1/4 teaspoon pepper
1/4 teaspoon dried thyme
1/2 teaspoon salt
2/3 cup uncooked long grain brown rice
1 medium onion, chopped
1 medium carrot, thinly sliced
1 tablespoon butter
1 tablespoon olive oil
2 pounds fresh asparagus, trimmed and cut into 1-inch pieces
6 cups reduced-sodium chicken broth
Reduced-fat sour cream

STEPS

1. In a 6-qt. stockpot, heat butter, and oil over medium heat. Stir in vegetables, salt, pepper, and thyme; cook, for 10 minutes, stirring occasionally.
2. Stir in rice and broth; bring to a boil. Reduce heat; simmer, covered, for 45 minutes, stirring occasionally.
3. Puree soup using an immersion blender. Return to pot and heat through.
4. Garnish with sour cream. Serve!

NUTRITION FACTS

Per Serving:
Calories: 79
Fat: 3 g
Saturated fat: 1 g
Carbohydrates: 11 g
Fiber: 2 g
Sodium: 401 mg
Cholesterol: 3 mg

Whole Grain Banana Pancakes

INGREDIENTS

1/2 teaspoon vanilla extract
1/2 teaspoon salt
1 teaspoon ground cinnamon
1 cup whole wheat flour
1 cup all-purpose flour
1 medium mashed ripe banana
1 tablespoon olive oil
1 tablespoon maple syrup
2 large eggs
2 cups fat-free milk
4 teaspoons baking powder
Sliced bananas and additional syrup

STEPS

1. Whisk together the whole wheat flour, all-purpose flour, baking powder, cinnamon, and salt. In another bowl, whisk milk, eggs, mashed banana, oil, 1 tablespoon syrup, and vanilla. Add to flour mixture; stir just until moistened.
2. Preheat a griddle coated with cooking spray over medium heat. Pour batter by 1/4 cupfuls onto griddle; cook until bubbles on top begin to pop and bottoms are golden brown. Turn; cook until the second side is golden brown.
3. Garnish with sliced bananas.
4. Serve!

NUTRITION FACTS

Per Serving:
Calories: 186
Fat: 4 g
Saturated fat: 1 g
Carbohydrates: 32 g
Fiber: 3 g
Sodium: 392 mg
Cholesterol: 48 mg

Almond Granola

INGREDIENTS

3/4 teaspoon salt
3/4 teaspoon ground cinnamon
3/4 teaspoon ground nutmeg
1/4 teaspoon ground cardamom
1/4 cup boiling water
1/4 cup olive oil
1/3 cup sugar
1/2 cup honey
1 cup sweetened shredded coconut
2 chai tea bags
2 cups almonds, coarsely chopped
2 teaspoons vanilla extract
3 cups quick-cooking oats

STEPS

1. Preheat oven to 250 degrees F. Steep tea bags in boiling water for 5 minutes. Meanwhile, combine oats, almonds, and coconut. Discard tea bags; stir the vanilla, salt, cinnamon, nutmeg, cardamom, olive oil, sugar, and honey into tea. Pour tea mixture over oat mixture; mix well to coat.
2. Spread evenly in a greased 15x10-in. rimmed pan. Bake, stirring every 20 minutes, about 1-1/4 hours.
3. Cool completely without stirring; store in an airtight container.
4. Serve!

NUTRITION FACTS

Per Serving:
Calories: 272
Fat: 16 g
Saturated fat: 3 g
Carbohydrates: 29 g
Fiber: 4 g
Sodium: 130 mg
Cholesterol: 0 mg

Black Bean & Sweet Potato Rice

INGREDIENTS

3/4 cup uncooked long grain rice
1/4 teaspoon garlic salt
1 large sweet potato, peeled and diced
1 medium red onion, finely chopped
1-1/2 cups water
2 tablespoons sweet chili sauce
3 tablespoons olive oil, divided
4 cups chopped fresh kale (tough stems removed)
15 ounces black beans, rinsed and drained
Lime wedges
Additional sweet chili sauce for garnish

STEPS

1. Place rice, garlic salt, and water in a saucepan; bring to a boil. Reduce heat; simmer, covered, for about 18 minutes. Remove from heat; let stand 5 minutes.
2. Meanwhile, in a skillet, heat 2 tablespoons oil over medium heat; saute sweet potato for 8 minutes. Add onion; cook and stir, for 6 minutes. Add kale; cook and stir, for 5 minutes. Stir in beans; heat through.
3. Gently stir 2 tablespoons chili sauce and remaining oil into rice; add to potato mixture.
4. Garnish with lime wedges and additional chili sauce. Serve!

NUTRITION FACTS

Per Serving:
Calories: 435
Fat: 11 g
Saturated fat: 2 g
Carbohydrates: 74 g
Fiber: 8 g
Sodium: 405 mg
Cholesterol: 0 g

Quark & Cucumber Toast

INGREDIENTS

1 slice whole-grain bread, toasted
1 tablespoon cilantro leaves
2 tablespoons quark
2 tablespoons diced cucumber
Pinch sea salt

STEPS

1. Top toast with quark, cucumber, cilantro and sea salt.
2. Serve!

NUTRITION FACTS

Per Serving:
Calories: 141
Fat: 5 g
Carbohydrates: 13 g
Fiber: 2 g
Protein: 7 g
Sodium: 300 mg
Cholesterol: 20 mg

Fish Tacos

INGREDIENTS

1/4 cup olive oil
1 cup chopped fresh cilantro
1 teaspoon ground cardamom
1 teaspoon paprika
1 teaspoon salt
1 teaspoon pepper
2 cups chopped red cabbage
2 medium limes, cut into wedges
6 mahi mahi fillets
12 corn tortillas
Salsa verde
Hot pepper sauce

STEPS

1. In a 13x9-in. baking dish, whisk the olive oil, cardamom, paprika, salt, and pepper. Add fillets; turn to coat. Refrigerate, covered, 20 minutes.
2. Drain fish and discard marinade. On an oiled grill rack, grill mahi-mahi, covered, over medium heat, for 5 minutes per side. Remove fish. Place tortillas on grill rack; heat for 50 seconds. Keep warm.
3. To assemble, divide fish among the tortillas; layer with red cabbage, cilantro and, salsa verde.
4. Squeeze a little lime juice and hot pepper sauce over fish mixture; fold sides of tortilla over the mixture. Serve with lime wedges and additional pepper sauce.

NUTRITION FACTS

Per Serving:
Calories: 284
Fat: 5 g
Saturated fat: 1 g
Carbohydrates: 26 g
Fiber: 4 g
Sodium: 278 mg
Cholesterol: 124 mg

SERVES FOR
8 PEOPLE

Chicken and Veggies Wraps

INGREDIENTS

1 cup frozen shelled edamame
DRESSING:
1/8 teaspoon pepper
1/4 teaspoon salt
1/2 teaspoon ground ginger
1 teaspoon sesame oil
2 tablespoons orange juice
2 tablespoons olive oil
WRAPS:
1/2 cup shredded carrots
1/2 cup thinly sliced sweet red pepper
1 cup thinly sliced cucumber
1 cup fresh sugar snap peas, chopped
1 cup chopped cooked chicken breast
2 cups fresh baby spinach
8 whole wheat tortillas, room temperature

STEPS

1. Cook edamame according to package directions. Drain; rinse with cold water and drain well. Whisk the sesame oil, olive oil, orange juice, ginger, salt, and pepper.
2. In a bowl, combine the carrots, sweet red pepper, cucumber, snap peans, chicken, spinach, chicken, and edamame; toss with the dressing. Place about 1/2 cup mixture on each tortilla. Fold bottom and sides of tortilla over filling and roll-up.
3. Serve!

NUTRITION FACTS

Per Serving:
Calories: 214
Fat: 7 g
Saturated fat: 1 g
Carbohydrates: 28 g
Fiber: 5 g
Sodium: 229 mg
Cholesterol: 13 mg

Tomato & Corn Pasta

INGREDIENTS

1/4 cup grated Parmesan cheese
1/2 teaspoon pepper
1/2 cup finely chopped red onion
1/2 cup part-skim ricotta cheese
1 cup fresh corn, thawed
1 teaspoon salt
1 teaspoon minced fresh rosemary, crushed
1 tablespoon olive oil
2 cups cherry tomatoes, halved
2 tablespoons minced fresh basil
3 garlic cloves, minced
3 cups baby spinach
12 ounces uncooked whole wheat elbow macaroni
15 ounces cannellini beans, rinsed and drained
Chopped fresh parsley

STEPS

1. Cook pasta according to package directions. Drain and rinse with cold water; drain well.
2. In a bowl, combine corn, tomatoes, beans, onion, ricotta, and Parmesan cheeses, oil, basil, garlic, rosemary, salt, and pepper. Stir in pasta.
3. Add baby spinach; toss gently to combine.
4. Garnish with parsley. Serve immediately!

NUTRITION FACTS

Per Serving:
Calories: 275
Fat: 5 g
Saturated fat: 1 g
Carbohydrates: 46 g
Fiber: 8 g
Sodium: 429 mg
Cholesterol: 7 mg

Corn Salad with Shrimp

INGREDIENTS

1/8 teaspoon pepper
1/4 cup olive oil
1/2 cup packed fresh basil leaves
1/2 teaspoon salt, divided
4 medium ears sweet corn, husked
1 medium ripe avocado, peeled and chopped
1 pound uncooked shrimp (31-40 per pound), peeled and deveined
1-1/2 cups cherry tomatoes, halved

STEPS

1. In a pot of boiling water, cook corn, for 6 minutes. Drain; cool slightly. Meanwhile, in a food processor, oil, pulse basil, and 1/4 teaspoon salt until blended.
2. Cut corn from cob and place in a bowl. Stir in tomatoes, pepper, and remaining salt. Add avocado and 2 tablespoons basil mixture; toss gently to combine.
3. Thread shrimp onto metal skewers; brush with remaining basil mixture. Grill, covered, over medium heat, for 4 minutes per side. Remove shrimp from skewers.
4. Serve with corn mixture!

NUTRITION FACTS

Per Serving:
Calories: 371
Fat: 22 g
Saturated fat: 3 g
Carbohydrates: 25 g
Fiber: 5 g
Sodium: 450 mg
Cholesterol: 138 mg

Grilled Beef Chimichangas

INGREDIENTS

1/4 teaspoon ground cumin
1/4 cup salsa
1 pound lean ground beef (90% lean)
1 small onion, chopped
2 garlic cloves, minced
3/4 cup shredded Monterey Jack cheese
4 ounces chopped green chiles
6 whole wheat tortillas
Reduced-fat sour cream and guacamole

STEPS

1. In a skillet, cook onion, garlic, and beef, over medium heat for 8 minutes, breaking up beef into crumbles; drain. Stir in chiles, salsa, and cumin.
2. Add 1/2 cup beef mixture across the center of each tortilla; garnish with 2 tablespoons cheese. Fold bottom and sides of tortilla over filling and roll-up.
3. Place chimichangas on grill rack, seam side down. Grill, covered, over low heat 13 minutes, turning once. Garnish with sour cream and guacamole.
4. Serve!

NUTRITION FACTS

Per Serving:
Calories: 295
Fat: 12 g
Carbohydrates: 25 g
Fiber: 4 g
Sodium: 370 mg
Protein: 22 g
Cholesterol: 60 mg

Breakfast Sweet Potatoes

INGREDIENTS

1/4 cup toasted unsweetened coconut flakes
1/2 cup fat-free coconut Greek yogurt
1 medium apple, chopped
2 tablespoons maple syrup
4 medium sweet potatoes

STEPS

1. Preheat oven to 425 degrees F. Place potatoes on a foil-lined baking sheet. Bake, for 60 minutes.
2. With a sharp knife, cut an "X" in each potato. Fluff pulp with a fork.
3. Garnish with coconut flakes, coconut Greek yogurt, apple, and maple syrup. Serve!

NUTRITION FACTS

Per Serving:
Calories: 321
Fat: 3 g
Saturated fat: 2 g
Carbohydrates: 70 g
Fiber: 8 g
Sodium: 36 mg
Cholesterol: 0 mg

Salmon with Pistachio Crust

INGREDIENTS

1/4 teaspoon crushed red pepper flakes
1/3 cup sour cream
1/2 teaspoon grated lemon zest
1/2 cup minced shallots
2/3 cup dry bread crumbs
2/3 cup chopped pistachios
1 tablespoon snipped fresh dill
1 garlic clove, minced
2 tablespoons olive oil
2 tablespoons prepared horseradish
6 salmon fillets

STEPS

1. Preheat oven to 375 degrees F. Place salmon, skin side down, in an ungreased 15x10x1-in. baking pan.
2. Spread sour cream over each fillet.
3. Combine the red pepper flakes, lemon zest, shallots, bread crumbs, pistachios, dill, clove, and olive oil. Pat crumb-nut mixture onto tops of salmon fillets, pressing to help coating adhere.
4. Bake for about 15 minutes.
5. Serve!

NUTRITION FACTS

Per Serving:
Calories: 376
Fat: 25 g
Saturated fat: 5 g
Carbohydrates: 15 g
Fiber: 2 g
Sodium: 219 mg
Cholesterol: 60 mg

Delicious Pork Salad

INGREDIENTS

1/2 teaspoon ground cumin
1/2 teaspoon dried oregano
1 boneless pork loin roast
1 teaspoon chili powder
1 teaspoon pepper
1 small red onion, chopped
1 cup fresh corn
1 cup crumbled part-skim mozzarella cheese
1-1/2 teaspoons salt
1-1/2 teaspoons hot pepper sauce
1-1/2 cups apple cider
2 medium tomatoes, chopped
3 garlic cloves, minced
4 ounces chopped green chiles, drained
12 cups torn mixed salad greens
15 ounces black beans, rinsed and drained

STEPS

1. Place pork in a 5- or 6-qt. slow cooker.
2. In a bowl, mix cider, garlic, green chiles, chili powder, pepper, cumin, salt, pepper sauce, and oregano; pour over pork. Cook, covered, on low for about 5 hours.
3. Remove roast from slow cooker; discard cooking juices.
4. Shred pork with 2 forks. Arrange salad greens on a large serving platter.
5. Garnish with black beans, pork, tomatoes, onion, corn, and cheese. Serve!

NUTRITION FACTS

Per Serving:
Calories: 233
Fat: 8 g
Saturated fat: 4 g
Carbohydrates: 12 g
Fiber: 3 g
Sodium: 321 mg
Cholesterol: 67 mg

Garlic Chicken and Mushrooms

INGREDIENTS

1/4 teaspoon pepper
1/2 teaspoon salt
1/2 cup dry white wine
1 tablespoon olive oil
1 medium onion, chopped
2 garlic cloves, minced
4 boneless skinless chicken breast halves
6 ounces sliced baby portobello mushrooms

STEPS

1. Pound chicken breasts with a meat mallet to 1/2-in. thickness; sprinkle with salt and pepper.
2. In a skillet, heat oil over medium heat; cook chicken for 6 minutes per side. Remove from pan; keep warm.
3. Add onion, and mushrooms to pan; cook and stir over medium-high heat, for about 3 minutes. Add garlic; cook and stir for 40 seconds. Add wine; bring to a boil, stirring to loosen browned bits from pan. Cook for 2 minutes.
4. Serve over chicken.

NUTRITION FACTS

Per Serving:
Calories: 243
Fat: 7 g
Saturated fat: 2 g
Carbohydrates: 5 g
Fiber: 1 g
Sodium: 381 mg
Cholesterol: 94 mg

Salad with Sesame and Ginger

INGREDIENTS

1/2 cup sesame ginger salad dressing
1/2 cup salted peanuts
1 cup fresh bean sprouts
2 green onions, diagonally sliced
5 ounces baby kale salad blend
3 clementines, peeled and segmented
10 ounces frozen shelled edamame, thawed
15 ounces garbanzo beans, rinsed and drained

STEPS

1. Divide salad blend among 6 bowls.
2. Garnish with peanuts, bean sprouts, kale, edamame, garbanzo beans, and clementines.
3. Serve with sesame ginger salad dressing.

NUTRITION FACTS

Per Serving:
Calories: 317
Fat: 17 g
Saturated fat: 2 g
Carbohydrates: 32 g
Fiber: 8 g
Sodium: 355 mg
Cholesterol: 0 mg

Shrimp and Lime Skewers

INGREDIENTS

1/4 teaspoon salt
1/4 teaspoon ground cumin
1/4 teaspoon pepper
1/3 cup chopped fresh cilantro
1/3 cup lime juice
1 pound uncooked shrimp (16-20 per pound), peeled and deveined
1 jalapeno pepper, seeded and minced
1-1/2 teaspoons grated lime zest
2 tablespoons olive oil
3 garlic cloves, minced
Lime slices

STEPS

1. Mix the olive oil, lime juice, lime zest, jalapeno pepper, cloves, cumin, cilantro, salt, and pepper; toss with shrimp. Let stand for 20 minutes.
2. Thread shrimp and lime slices onto 4 metal skewers.
3. Grill, covered, over medium heat, for 4 minutes per side.
4. Serve!

NUTRITION FACTS

Per Serving:
Calories: 167
Fat: 8 g
Saturated fat: 1 g
Carbohydrates: 4 g
Fiber: 0 g
Sodium: 284 mg
Cholesterol: 138 mg

Creamy Lentils with Artichoke

INGREDIENTS

1/8 teaspoon pepper
1/4 teaspoon sea salt, divided
1/4 teaspoon dried oregano
1/2 teaspoon Italian seasoning
1/2 cup dried red lentils, rinsed and sorted
1 tablespoon olive oil
1-1/4 cups vegetable broth
2 tablespoons grated Romano cheese
2 cups hot cooked brown
3 garlic cloves, minced
12 ounces chopped fresh kale
14 ounces water-packed artichoke hearts, drained and chopped

STEPS

1. Place the vegetable broth, red lentils, oregano, pepper, and 1/8 teaspoon salt in a saucepan; bring to a boil. Reduce heat; simmer, covered, for about 15 minutes. Remove from heat.
2. In a 6-qt. stockpot, heat oil over medium heat. Add kale and remaining salt; cook, covered, for 5 minutes, stirring occasionally. Add artichoke hearts, garlic, and Italian seasoning; cook and stir for 4 minutes. Remove from heat; stir in cheese.
3. Serve lentils and kale mixture over rice.

NUTRITION FACTS

Per Serving:
Calories: 321
Fat: 6 g
Saturated fat: 2 g
Carbohydrates: 53 g
Fiber: 5 g
Sodium: 661 mg
Cholesterol: 1 mg

Quinoa and Peppers

INGREDIENTS

3/4 cup chopped sweet onion
3/4 cup quinoa, rinsed
1/8 teaspoon salt
1/4 teaspoon pepper
1/4 teaspoon garam masala
1-1/2 cups vegetable stock
1 pound Italian turkey sausage links, casings removed
1 medium sweet red pepper, chopped
1 medium green pepper, chopped
1 garlic clove, minced

STEPS

1. In a saucepan, bring the stock to a boil. Add quinoa. Reduce heat; simmer, covered, for about 15 minutes. Remove from heat.
2. In a skillet, cook onion and crumble sausage with peppers over medium heat, for 8 minutes.
3. Add garlic and seasonings; cook and stir for 1 minute. Stir in quinoa.
4. Serve!

NUTRITION FACTS

Per Serving:
Calories: 261
Fat: 9 g
Saturated fat: 2 g
Carbohydrates: 28 g
Fiber: 4 g
Sodium: 760 mg
Cholesterol: 42 mg

White Beans & Pasta

INGREDIENTS

3/4 teaspoon freshly ground pepper
1/2 cup crumbled feta cheese
1 tablespoon olive oil
1 medium zucchini, sliced
2 garlic cloves, minced
2 large tomatoes, chopped
2-1/4 ounces sliced ripe olives, drained
6 ounces uncooked whole wheat bow tie pasta
15 ounces cannellini beans, rinsed and drained

STEPS

1. Cook pasta according to package directions. Drain, reserving 1/2 cup pasta water.
2. Meanwhile, in a skillet, heat oil over medium heat; saute zucchini, for about 4 minutes. Add garlic; cook and stir for 40 seconds. Stir in beans, tomatoes, olives, and pepper; bring to a boil. Reduce heat; simmer, uncovered, for 5 minutes, stirring occasionally.
3. Stir in pasta and enough pasta water to moisten as desired.
4. Garnish with cheese. Serve!

NUTRITION FACTS

Per Serving:
Calories: 348
Fat: 9 g
Saturated fat: 2 g
Carbohydrates: 52 g
Fiber: 11 g
Sodium: 394 mg
Cholesterol: 8 mg

Chickpea Curry

INGREDIENTS

3/4 teaspoon salt
1/2 teaspoon ground turmeric
1 medium serrano pepper, cut into thirds
1 medium yellow onion, chopped
1 piece fresh ginger, peeled and coarsely chopped
2 teaspoons garam masala
2 teaspoons ground coriander
2 teaspoons ground cumin
2 1/4 cups no-salt-added canned diced tomatoes with their juice
4 large cloves garlic
6 tablespoons canola oil
15-ounce chickpeas, rinsed
Fresh cilantro for garnish

STEPS

1. Pulse garlic, serrano, and ginger in a food processor until minced. Scrape down the sides and pulse again. Add onion; pulse until finely chopped.
2. Heat oil in a saucepan over medium heat. Add the onion mixture and cook, stirring occasionally, for about 5 minutes. Add coriander, turmeric, cumin, and cook, stirring, for 2 minutes.
3. Pulse tomatoes in the food processor until finely chopped. Add to the pan along with salt. Reduce heat to maintain a simmer and cook, stirring occasionally, for 4 minutes. Add chickpeas and garam masala, reduce heat to a gentle simmer, cover, and cook, for 5 minutes more.
4. Garnish with cilantro. Serve!

NUTRITION FACTS

Per Serving:

Calories: 278
Fat: 15 g
Saturated fat: 1.2 g
Carbohydrates: 30 g
Fiber: 6.3 g
Sodium: 354 mg

Salad with Salmon & Sauce Garlic

INGREDIENTS

1/4 teaspoon ground pepper
1/4 cup mayonnaise
1/2 cup low-fat plain yogurt
1/2 cup sunflower seeds, toasted
1 pound salmon fillet
1 medium clove garlic, minced
1 tablespoon finely chopped fresh parsley
1 tablespoon snipped fresh chives
2 tablespoons lemon juice
2 tablespoons grated Parmesan cheese
2 teaspoons reduced-sodium soy sauce
2 cups chopped broccoli
2 cups chopped red cabbage
2 cups finely diced carrots
8 cups chopped curly kale

STEPS

1. Preheat broiler to high. Arrange a rack in the upper third of the oven. Line a baking sheet with foil.
2. Place salmon on the prepared baking sheet, skin-side down. Broil, rotating the pan from front to back once, for 12 minutes. Cut into 4 portions.
3. Meanwhile, whisk yogurt, lemon juice, soy sauce, garlic, mayonnaise, Parmesan, parsley, chives, and pepper in a bowl.
4. Combine kale, cabbage, broccoli, carrots, and sunflower seeds in another bowl. Add 3/4 cup of the dressing and toss to coat. Divide the salad among 4 dinner plates and garnish each with a piece of salmon and about 1 tablespoon of the remaining dressing.
5. Serve!

NUTRITION FACTS

Per Serving:
Calories: 409
Fat: 24 g
Saturated fat: 4 g
Carbohydrates: 18 g
Fiber: 6 g
Sodium: 356 mg
Cholesterol: 62 mg

Couscous with Chicken & Vegetables

INGREDIENTS

1/4 cup toasted sliced almonds
1/4 cup crumbled reduced-fat feta cheese
1/4 cup tahini
1/4 cup water
1/4 teaspoon ground pepper
1/4 teaspoon crushed red pepper
1/2 medium red bell pepper, chopped
1/2 teaspoon salt
1 cup whole-wheat pearl couscous
1 clove garlic, minced
1 tablespoon chopped fresh parsley
1 lemon, cut into wedges
2 teaspoons lemon zest
2 tablespoons lemon juice
2 tablespoons olive oil, divided
2 cups sliced mushrooms
4 cups coleslaw mix
4 cups baby spinach
12 ounces cooked chicken breast, chopped

NUTRITION FACTS

Per Serving:
Calories: 258
Fat: 23 g
Saturated fat: 4 g
Carbohydrates: 41 g
Fiber: 9 g
Sodium: 565 mg
Cholesterol: 77 mg

STEPS

1. Cook couscous in a saucepan according to package directions. Fluff with a fork and set aside.
2. Meanwhile, whisk tahini, 1 Tbsp. oil, water, lemon juice, salt, pepper, and crushed red pepper in a bowl until well blended; set aside.
3. Heat the remaining 1 Tbsp. oil in a nonstick skillet over medium heat. Add garlic and cook, for 40 seconds. Add mushrooms and bell pepper; cook, for 4 minutes.
4. Stir in coleslaw mix and spinach; continue cooking, stirring, for 3 minutes. Stir in couscous, chicken, and the tahini sauce; cook, for 5 minutes.
5. Garnish with feta, almonds, parsley, and lemon zest.
6. Serve with lemon wedges.

Stuffed Cucumbers

INGREDIENTS

1/2 cup fat-free plain Greek yogurt
1/2 teaspoon garlic salt
1/2 cup fresh peas, thawed
1 cup chopped cooked chicken breast
1 cup chopped seeded tomato, divided
2 tablespoons mayonnaise
2 medium cucumbers
3 teaspoons snipped fresh dill, divided

STEPS

1. Cut each cucumber lengthwise in half; scoop out pulp, leaving a 1/4-in. shell. In a bowl, mix mayonnaise, yogurt, garlic salt, and 1 teaspoon dill; gently stir in chicken, 3/4 cup tomato, and peas.
2. Spoon into cucumber shells.
3. Top with the remaining tomato and dill.
4. Serve!

NUTRITION FACTS

Per Serving:
Calories: 312
Fat: 12 g
Carbohydrates: 18 g
Fiber: 6 g
Protein: 34 g
Sodium: 641 mg
Cholesterol: 55 mg

Deliciuos Summer Salad

INGREDIENTS

3/4 teaspoon salt, divided
1/2 cup plus 2 tablespoons low-fat buttermilk
1 small garlic clove
1 cup chopped fresh parsley, and cilantro
1 cup lightly packed microgreens
1 cup fresh corn kernels
1 cup frozen edamame, thawed
1 small watermelon radish, halved and thinly sliced on a mandoline
2 tablespoons extra-virgin olive oil
2 small ripe avocados
2 tablespoons water
2 tablespoons plus 4 teaspoons fresh lemon juice, divided
3 small golden beets, peeled and trimmed
8 cups chopped romaine lettuce
15.5 ounce no-salt-added chickpeas, drained and rinsed

NUTRITION FACTS

Per Serving:
Calories: 292
Fat: 15 g
Saturated fat: 2 g
Carbohydrates: 30 g
Fiber: 10 g
Sodium: 400 mg
Cholesterol: 1 mg

STEPS

1. Wrap beets together in 1 sheet of microwavable parchment paper. Microwave on High, for about 12 minutes. Let cool for 5 minutes. Cut each beet into 8 wedges.
2. Meanwhile, cut 1 avocado into 12 wedges. Chop the remaining avocado.
3. Combine herbs, buttermilk, water, garlic, 2 tablespoons plus 2 teaspoons lemon juice, and 1/4 teaspoon salt in a blender. Puree until smooth, about 15 seconds. Add the chopped avocado; process on medium speed, for about 20 seconds.
4. Arrange romaine on a large platter. Top with microgreens, corn, beet wedges, chickpeas, edamame, radish slices, and avocado wedges. Sprinkle with oil, the remaining 2 teaspoons lemon juice, and the remaining 1/2 teaspoon salt. Spoon the buttermilk dressing over the salad. Serve!

Creamy Pasta with Shrimp and Lemon

INGREDIENTS

1/4 cup thinly sliced fresh basil
1/4 cup whole-milk plain yogurt
1/4 teaspoon crushed red pepper
1/4 teaspoon salt
1/3 cup grated Parmesan cheese, plus more for garnish
1 tablespoon extra-virgin olive oil
1 teaspoon lemon zest
1 tablespoon finely chopped garlic
2 tablespoons lemon juice
2 tablespoons unsalted butter
4 cups loosely packed arugula
8 ounces whole-wheat fettuccine
12 ounces sustainably sourced peeled and deveined raw shrimp (26-30 per pound)

NUTRITION FACTS

Per Serving:
Calories: 403
Fat: 13 g
Saturated fat: 5 g
Carbohydrates: 45 g
Fiber: 6 g
Sodium: 396 mg
Cholesterol: 159 mg

STEPS

1. Bring 7 cups of water to a boil. Add fettuccine, stirring to separate the noodles. Cook, for 10 minutes. Reserve 1/2 cup of the cooking water and drain.
2. Meanwhile, heat oil in a nonstick skillet over medium heat. Add shrimp and cook, stirring occasionally, for 3 minutes. Transfer the shrimp to a bowl.
3. Add butter to the pan and reduce heat. Add garlic and crushed red pepper; cook, stirring often, about 1 minute. Add arugula and cook, stirring, for about 1 minute. Reduce heat to low. Add the fettuccine, lemon zest, yogurt, and the reserved cooking water, 1/4 cup at a time, tossing well, until the fettuccine is fully coated and creamy. Add the shrimp, lemon juice, and salt, tossing to coat the fettuccine. Remove from the heat and toss with Parmesan.
4. Garnish with basil and more Parmesan. Serve!

Chicken & Chickpea Soup

INGREDIENTS

1/4 cup chopped fresh parsley
1/4 cup halved pitted oil-cured olives
1/4 teaspoon cayenne pepper
1/4 teaspoon ground pepper
1/2 teaspoon salt
1 bay leaf
1 large yellow onion, finely chopped
1 1/2 cups dried chickpeas, soaked overnight
2 tablespoons tomato paste
2 pounds bone-in chicken thighs, skin removed, trimmed
4 cups water
4 cloves garlic, finely chopped
4 teaspoons ground cumin
4 teaspoons paprika
14 ounce artichoke hearts, drained and quartered
15 ounce no-salt-added diced tomatoes, preferably fire-roasted

STEPS

1. Drain chickpeas and place them in a 6-quart slow cooker. Add 4 cups water, onion, garlic, bay leaf, tomatoes and their juice, tomato paste, paprika, cumin, cayenne, and ground pepper; stir to combine. Add chicken.
2. Cover and cook on High for 4 hours.
3. Transfer the chicken to a cutting board and let cool slightly. Discard bay leaf. Add olives, artichokes, and salt to the slow cooker and stir to combine. Shred the chicken, discarding bones. Stir the chicken into the soup.
4. Garnish with parsley. Serve!

NUTRITION FACTS

Per Serving:
Calories: 447
Fat: 15 g
Saturated fat: 3 g
Carbohydrates: 43 g
Fiber: 11 g
Sodium: 761 mg
Cholesterol: 76 mg

Eggplant Parmesan

INGREDIENTS

1/4 cup prepared pesto
1/2 cup whole-wheat panko bread-crumbs
1 tablespoon chopped fresh basil
1 cup prepared low-sodium marinara sauce
2 tablespoons extra-virgin olive oil plus 2 teaspoons, divided
2 tablespoons grated Parmesan cheese
4 ounces fresh mozzarella, thinly sliced into 12 pieces
4 small eggplants

STEPS

1. Preheat oven to 400 degrees F.
2. Spread sauce in a broiler-safe baking dish. Make crosswise cuts every 1/4 inch of each eggplant, slicing almost to the bottom but not all the way through. Carefully transfer the eggplants to the baking dish. Gently fan them to open the cuts wider. Sprinkle 2 tablespoons of oil over the eggplants. Fill the cuts alternately with mozzarella and pesto. Cover with foil.
3. Bake, for about 50 minutes.
4. Combine Parmesan, panko, and the remaining 2 teaspoons of oil in a bowl. Remove the foil and sprinkle the eggplants with the breadcrumb mixture.
5. Increase the oven temperature to broil. Broil the eggplants on the center rack until the topping is golden brown, for 4 minutes.
6. Garnish with basil. Serve with the sauce.

NUTRITION FACTS

Per Serving:
Calories: 349
Fat: 22 g
Saturated fat: 6 g
Carbohydrates: 24 g
Fiber: 7 g
Sodium: 405 mg
Cholesterol: 25 mg

Chocolate Smoothie With Avocado

INGREDIENTS

1/4 cup unsweetened cocoa powder
1/2 avocado, pitted and peeled
1 medium banana, peeled
2 cups vanilla soy milk
2 individual packets Splenda

STEPS

1. Place cocoa powder, avocado, banana, vanilla soy milk, and Splenda in a blender and process until smooth.
2. Serve immediately!

NUTRITION FACTS

Per Serving:
Calories: 252
Fat: 12 g
Saturated fat: 2 g
Carbohydrates: 33 g
Fiber: 8 g
Sodium: 102 mg
Cholesterol: 0 mg

Tuna and Spinach Sandwiches

INGREDIENTS

1/4 teaspoon freshly ground black pepper
1/2 teaspoon salt-free seasoning blend
1/2 small red onion, peeled and diced
1/2 teaspoon dill weed
1/2 medium cucumber, peeled, seeded, and diced
1 cup fresh baby spinach
2 ribs celery, diced
2 tablespoons olive oil
6.4-ounce tuna packed in water
8 slices whole-wheat bread
Juice of one lemon

STEPS

1. Combine the cucumber, onion, celery, tuna, and dill weed.
2. Sprinkle with olive oil and lemon juice, and stir. Season with salt-free seasoning blend and pepper.
3. Make the sandwich with 1/2 cup tuna salad and 1/4 cup baby spinach leaves. Press down to compact the tuna and the spinach.
4. Serve!

NUTRITION FACTS

Per Serving:
Calories: 192
Fat: 3 g
Saturated fat: 1 g
Carbohydrates: 27 g
Fiber: 4 g
Sodium: 450 mg
Cholesterol: 14 mg

Italian-Style Roasted Salmon

INGREDIENTS

1/4 cup minced fresh dill
1 lemon, cut into 4 wedges
4 wild salmon fillets
4 cloves garlic, peeled and minced
Freshly ground black pepper

STEPS

1. Preheat oven to 425 degrees F. Coat a glass baking dish with nonstick cooking spray. Place the salmon fillets in the baking dish.
2. Squeeze juice from one wedge of lemon over each fillet.
3. Sprinkle the salmon with black pepper, dill, and garlic.
4. Bake, for about 20 minutes.
5. Serve!

NUTRITION FACTS

Per Serving:
Calories: 251
Fat: 11 g
Saturated fat: 2 g
Carbohydrates: 2 g
Fiber: 1 g
Sodium: 78 mg
Cholesterol: 94 mg

Spicy Roasted Broccoli

INGREDIENTS

1/4 teaspoon crushed red pepper flakes
1/4 teaspoon freshly ground black pepper
1/2 teaspoon salt-free seasoning blend
4 tablespoons olive oil, divided
4 cloves garlic, peeled and minced
8 cups broccoli, large stems trimmed and cut into 2-inch pieces

STEPS

1. Preheat the oven to 450 degrees F.
2. In a bowl, toss the broccoli and 2 tablespoons of olive oil.
3. Sprinkle with salt-free seasoning and pepper. Transfer to a rimmed baking sheet and bake for 14 minutes.
4. Meanwhile, mix together 2 tablespoons of olive oil, garlic, and red pepper flakes.
5. After the broccoli has cooked for 14 minutes, sprinkle the garlic oil over the broccoli and toss to coat the broccoli.
6. Return to the oven and continue baking for 10 more minutes.
7. Serve hot!

NUTRITION FACTS

Per Serving:
Calories: 86
Fat: 7 g
Saturated fat: 1 g
Carbohydrates: 5 g
Fiber: 2 g
Sodium: 24 mg
Cholesterol: 0 mg

Garlic Mashed Potatoes

INGREDIENTS

1/4 cup olive oil
1/2 teaspoon freshly ground black pepper
1 teaspoon salt-free seasoning blend
2 pounds all-purpose gold potatoes, scrubbed and cut into large chunks
6 cloves garlic, peeled

STEPS

1. Place the potato chunks and peeled garlic cloves in a saucepan. Cover with cold water and bring to a boil.
2. Reduce the heat and cook for about 35 minutes.
3. Remove from heat.
4. Drain the cooking liquid off the potatoes, reserving 3/4 cup of the cooking liquid.
5. Add the olive oil, salt-free seasoning blend, pepper, and reserved cooking liquid to the potatoes.
6. Mash with a potato masher.
7. Taste and season with more salt-free seasoning and pepper. Serve!

NUTRITION FACTS

Per Serving:
Calories: 145
Fat: 7 g
Saturated fat: 1 g
Carbohydrates: 19 g
Fiber: 2 g
Sodium: 7 mg
Cholesterol: 0 mg

Avocado Toast

INGREDIENTS

1/4 medium avocado, mashed
1 slice whole-grain bread, toasted
2 teaspoons everything bagel seasoning
Pinch of flaky sea salt

STEPS

1. Spread avocado on toast.
2. Garnish with seasoning and
   salt.

NUTRITION FACTS

Per Serving:

Calories: 172
Fat: 9.8 g
Carbohydrates: 17.8 g
Fiber: 5.9 g
Protein: 5.4 g
Sodium: 251 mg

Porridge Bowl

INGREDIENTS

1/2 cup milk
1/2 banana, sliced
1 orange, 1/2 sliced and 1/2 juiced
1 tbsp goji berries
1 tbsp chia seeds
2 tbsp smooth almond butter
4 oz. frozen raspberries
5 oz. porridge oats

STEPS

1. Tip half the raspberries and all of the orange juice in a pan. Simmer, for 5 mins.
2. Meanwhile stir the oats, milk, and 2 cups water in a pan over low heat until creamy.
3. Garnish with the orange slices, raspberry compote, remaining raspberries, banana, almond butter, goji berries, and chia seeds. Serve!

NUTRITION FACTS

Per Serving:

Calories: 533
Fat: 19 g
Saturated fat: 3 g
Carbohydrates: 66 g
Fiber: 13 g
Sodium: 0.1 g

Eggplant & Tomato Pasta

INGREDIENTS

1/4 teaspoon crushed red pepper
1/4 cup shaved crumbled feta cheese
1/2 cup chopped fresh basil
1/2 teaspoon salt
1/2 teaspoon ground pepper
1 clove garlic, grated
1 pound plum tomatoes, chopped
1 1/2 pounds eggplant, cut into 1/2-inch-thick slices
2 teaspoons chopped fresh oregano
4 tablespoons extra-virgin olive oil, divided
8 ounces whole-wheat penne

STEPS

1. Put a pot of water on to boil. Preheat grill to medium-high.
2. Toss tomatoes with 3 tablespoons oil, garlic, crushed red pepper, oregano, pepper, and salt in a bowl.
3. Brush eggplant with the remaining 1 tablespoon oil. Grill, turning once, for 5 minutes per side. Let cool for 5 minutes. Chop into bite-size pieces and add to the tomatoes along with basil.
4. Meanwhile, cook pasta according to package directions. Drain.
5. Serve the tomato mixture on the pasta.
6. Garnish with cheese. Serve!

NUTRITION FACTS

Per Serving:
Calories: 449
Fat: 19 g
Saturated fat: 3 g
Carbohydrates: 62 g
Fiber: 12 g
Sodium: 392 mg
Cholesterol: 8 mg

Soup Chickpea & Potato Curry

INGREDIENTS

3/4 cup water, divided
3/4 teaspoon salt
1/4 teaspoon cayenne pepper
1/2 teaspoon garam masala
1 pound potatoes, peeled and cut into 1-inch pieces
1 large onion, diced
1 cup frozen peas
2 teaspoons curry powder
3 tablespoons canola oil
3 cloves garlic, minced
14 ounce no-salt-added diced tomatoes
15 ounce low-sodium chickpeas, rinsed

NUTRITION FACTS

Per Serving:

Calories: 321
Fat: 11 g
Saturated fat: 1 g
Carbohydrates: 46 g
Fiber: 9 g
Sodium: 532 mg

STEPS

1. Bring 1 inch of water to a boil in a pot fitted with a steamer basket. Add potatoes, cover, and steam, for 8 minutes. Set the potatoes aside. Dry the pot.
2. Heat oil in the pot over medium heat. Add onion and cook, stirring often, for about 5 minutes. Add garlic, curry powder, salt, and cayenne; cook, stirring constantly, for 1 minute. Stir in tomatoes and their juice; cook for 3 minutes. Transfer the mixture to a blender. Add 1/2 cup water and puree until smooth.
3. Return the puree to the pot. Pulse the remaining 1/4 cup water in the blender to rinse the sauce residue. Add to the pot along with the reserved potatoes, chickpeas, peas, and garam masala. Cook, stirring often, for 6 minutes.
4. Serve!

Pineapple Cream

INGREDIENTS

1 tablespoon lemon juice
1 large mango, peeled, seeded, and chopped
16 ounce frozen pineapple chunks

STEPS

1. Process mango, pineapple, and lemon juice in a food processor until smooth and creamy.
2. For the best texture, serve immediately!

NUTRITION FACTS

Per Serving:

Calories: 55
Fat: 0.2 g
Carbohydrates: 14.2 g
Fiber: 1.5 g
Protein: 0.6 g
Sodium: 1.1 mg

Potatoes with Salsa & Beans

INGREDIENTS

1/2 cup fresh salsa
1 ripe avocado, sliced
4 teaspoons chopped pickled jalapeños
4 medium russet potatoes
15 ounce pinto beans, rinsed, warmed and lightly mashed

STEPS

1. Pierce potatoes all over with a fork. Microwave on Medium, turning once, for 20 minutes. Transfer to a cutting board and let cool slightly.
2. Holding them with a kitchen towel to protect your hands, make a lengthwise cut to open the potato, but don't cut all the way through. Pinch the ends to expose the flesh.
3. Garnish each potato with some salsa, avocado, beans, and jalapeños. Serve warm!

NUTRITION FACTS

Per Serving:

Calories: 324
Fat: 8 g
Saturated fat: 1 g
Carbohydrates: 56 g
Fiber: 11 g
Sodium: 421 mg

Chickpea & Quinoa Salad

INGREDIENTS

1/4 avocado, diced
1/3 cup canned chickpeas, rinsed and drained
1/2 cup cucumber slices
1/2 cup cherry tomatoes, halved
1 cup cooked quinoa
1 tablespoon finely chopped roasted red pepper
1 tablespoon lemon juice
1 tablespoon water
1 teaspoon chopped fresh parsley
3 tablespoons hummus
Pinch of salt
Pinch of ground pepper

STEPS

1. Arrange chickpeas, cucumbers, quinoa, tomatoes, and avocado in a bowl.
2. Stir roasted red pepper, hummus, lemon juice, and water in the bowl with the chickpeas.
3. Add parsley, salt, and pepper and stir to combine.
4. Serve!

NUTRITION FACTS

Per Serving:

Calories: 503
Fat: 16 g
Saturated fat: 2 g
Carbohydrates: 75 g
Fiber: 16 g
Sodium: 572 mg

Vegetable Soup

INGREDIENTS

1/4 teaspoon salt
1/2 cup all-purpose flour
1 cup whole milk
1 cup diced onion
1 cup diced celery
1 tablespoon chili powder
1 1/2 teaspoons ground cumin
1 teaspoon dried oregano
2 cups diced sweet potato
2 medium red bell peppers, diced
3 tablespoons extra-virgin olive oil
4 cups reduced-sodium vegetable broth
15 ounce black beans, rinsed
Cilantro for garnish
Toasted pepitas for garnish
Lime wedges for garnish

STEPS

1. Heat oil in a pot over medium heat. Add onion and celery; cook, stirring frequently for 6 minutes. Sprinkle flour, chili powder, oregano, cumin, and salt over the vegetables and cook, stirring, for 1 minute more. Add vegetable broth and milk; bring to a gentle boil, stirring constantly.
2. Stir in sweet potatoes and peppers and bring just to a simmer. Simmer, uncovered, stirring occasionally, for 15 minutes.
3. Add black beans and cook, stirring frequently, for 5 minutes.
4. Garnish with lime wedges.
5. Serve topped with cilantro and pepitas.

NUTRITION FACTS

Per Serving:
Calories: 307
Fat: 10 g
Saturated fat: 1 g
Carbohydrates: 43 g
Fiber: 10 g
Sodium: 310 mg
Cholesterol: 4 mg

Vegetable & Egg Scramble

INGREDIENTS

1/2 teaspoon salt

1 teaspoon minced fresh herbs, such as rosemary

2 tablespoons olive oil

2 cups packed leafy greens, such as baby spinach

3 scallions, thinly sliced, green and white parts separated

4 cups thinly sliced vegetables, such as mushrooms, bell peppers, and zucchini

6 large eggs, lightly beaten

12 ounces baby potatoes, thinly sliced

STEPS

1. Heat oil in a nonstick skillet over medium heat. Add potatoes; cover and cook, stirring several times for 10 minutes.
2. Add sliced vegetables and scallion whites; cook uncovered, stirring occasionally, for 10 minutes. Stir in herbs. Move the vegetable mixture to the perimeter of the pan.
3. Reduce heat to low. Add eggs and scallion greens to the center of the pan. Cook, stirring for 3 minutes.
4. Stir leafy greens into the eggs. Remove from heat and stir to combine well add in salt.
5. Serve!

NUTRITION FACTS

Per Serving:
Calories: 254
Fat: 14 g
Saturated fat: 3 g
Carbohydrates: 19 g
Fiber: 4 g
Sodium: 415 mg
Cholesterol: 279 mg

Vegetarian Pasta

INGREDIENTS

28 ounce diced tomatoes
1/2 cup dry white wine
1/2 cup low-sodium vegetable broth
1 cup chopped onion
1/2 cup chopped celery
1/2 cup chopped carrot
3 tablespoons extra-virgin olive oil
2 tablespoons minced garlic
1 teaspoon Italian seasoning
1/2 teaspoon salt
1/4 teaspoon ground pepper
15 ounce cans no-salt-added cannellini beans, rinsed
1/4 cup heavy cream
1 pound whole-wheat spaghetti
1/2 cup grated Parmesan cheese
1/4 cup chopped fresh basil

STEPS

1. Combine oil, onion, garlic, carrot, celery, tomatoes, wine, broth, Italian seasoning, salt, and pepper in a 5-quart slow cooker. Cook on High for 3 hours. Stir in beans and cream at the end of the cooking time. Keep warm.
2. Meanwhile, bring a pot of water to a boil. Cook spaghetti according to package directions; drain.
3. Garnish with the sauce, Parmesan, and basil. Serve!

NUTRITION FACTS

Per Serving:
Calories: 434
Fat: 12 g
Saturated fat: 3 g
Carbohydrates: 64 g
Fiber: 7 g
Sodium: 411 mg
Cholesterol: 12 mg

Mexican Black Bean Salad

INGREDIENTS

1/4 cup cilantro leaves
1/4 cup lime juice
1/2 teaspoon salt
1/2 cup thinly sliced red onion
1 medium ripe avocado, pitted and roughly chopped
1 clove garlic, minced
1 pint grape tomatoes, halved
2 tablespoons extra-virgin olive oil
2 cups frozen corn, thawed and patted dry
8 cups mixed salad greens
15 ounce mexican black beans, rinsed

STEPS

1. Place onion in a bowl and cover with cold water. Set aside. Combine oil, lime juice, avocado, garlic, cilantro, and salt in a mini food processor. Process, scraping down the sides as needed, until smooth and creamy.
2. Just before serving, combine salad greens, tomatoes, corn, and beans in a bowl. Drain the onions and add to the bowl, along with the avocado dressing.
3. Serve!

NUTRITION FACTS

Per Serving:

Calories: 322
Fat: 16 g
Saturated fat: 2 g
Carbohydrates: 40 g
Fiber: 12 g
Sodium: 406 mg

Stuffed Sweet Potato

INGREDIENTS

3/4 cup chopped kale
1/4 cup hummus
1 cup canned black beans, rinsed
1 large sweet potato, scrubbed
2 tablespoons water

STEPS

1. Prick sweet potato all over with a fork. Microwave on High for 10 minutes.
2. Meanwhile, wash kale and drain, allowing water to cling to the leaves. Place in a saucepan; cover and cook over medium heat, stirring once, until wilted. Add beans; add a tablespoon of water if the pot is dry. Continue cooking, uncovered, stirring occasionally, for 2 minutes.
3. Split the sweet potato open and top with the kale and bean mixture. Combine hummus and 2 tablespoons of water in a dish.
4. Garnish the hummus dressing over the stuffed sweet potato. Serve!

NUTRITION FACTS

Per Serving:

Calories: 472
Fat: 7 g
Saturated fat: 1 g
Carbohydrates: 85 g
Fiber: 22 g
Sodium: 489 mg

Veggies & Black Bean Tacos

INGREDIENTS

1/4 teaspoon salt
1/4 teaspoon ground pepper
1/2 teaspoon ground coriander
1/2 avocado, cut into 8 slices
1/2 cup cooked black beans, rinsed
1 cup roasted root vegetables
1 teaspoon ground cumin
1 teaspoon chili powder
1 lime, cut into wedges
2 teaspoons extra-virgin olive oil
4 corn tortillas, lightly toasted
Chopped fresh cilantro & salsa for garnish

STEPS

1. Combine the oil, roasted root vegetables, beans, chili powder, cumin, coriander, salt, and pepper in a saucepan.
2. Cover and cook over medium heat for 8 minutes.
3. Divide the mixture among the tortillas and add avocado.
4. Garnish with cilantro and salsa.
5. Serve with lime wedges.

NUTRITION FACTS

Per Serving:

Calories: 343
Fat: 16 g
Saturated fat: 2 g
Carbohydrates: 44 g
Fiber: 12 g
Sodium: 352 mg

Bowls with Bean & Pumpkin

INGREDIENTS

3/4 teaspoon salt
1/4 teaspoon cayenne pepper
1 teaspoon ground cinnamon
1 tablespoon extra-virgin olive oil
1 1/2 cups chopped carrot
2 teaspoons ground cumin
3 large cloves garlic, minced
3 cups chopped onion
3 tablespoons chili powder
4 cups low-sodium vegetable broth
3 cups diced pumpkin squash
15-ounce low-sodium black beans, rinsed
28 ounce no-salt-added crushed tomatoes
Diced onion, sliced jalapeños, Cotija cheese and pepitas for garnish

STEPS

1. Heat oil in a pot over medium heat. Add onion and cook, stirring often, for about 5 minutes.
2. Reduce heat to low, add carrot and continue cooking, stirring often, for 5 minutes more.
3. Add garlic and cook, stirring, for 1 minute.
4. Stir in broth, scraping up any browned bits, and bring to a boil over high heat.
5. Add pumpkin, beans, tomatoes, cinnamon, cumin, chili powder, salt, and cayenne. Cover and return to a boil.
6. Reduce heat to maintain a gentle simmer and cook, uncovered, for 40 minutes.
7. Serve garnished with onion, cheese, jalapeños, and pepitas.

NUTRITION FACTS

Per Serving:

Calories: 276
Fat: 2 g
Saturated fat: 0.4 g
Carbohydrates: 49 g
Fiber: 16 g
Sodium: 508 mg

Chicken Thighs with Peppers & Potatoes

INGREDIENTS

1/4 teaspoon pepper
1/2 teaspoon salt
2 pounds red potatoes
2 large sweet red peppers
2 large green peppers
2 medium onions
2 tablespoons olive oil, divided
3 teaspoons minced fresh rosemary, crushed, divided
4 teaspoons minced fresh thyme, divided
8 boneless skinless chicken thighs

STEPS

1. Preheat oven to 450 degrees F.
2. Cut potatoes, peppers, and onions into 1-in. pieces.
3. Place vegetables in a roasting pan. Drizzle with 1 tablespoon oil; sprinkle with 2 teaspoons each thyme and rosemary and toss to coat. Place chicken over vegetables. Brush chicken with remaining oil; sprinkle with remaining thyme and rosemary.
4. Drizzle vegetables and chicken with salt and pepper.
5. Roast for 40 minutes. Serve!

NUTRITION FACTS

Per Serving:
Calories: 308
Fat: 12 g
Saturated fat: 3 g
Carbohydrates: 25 g
Fiber: 4 g
Sodium: 221 mg
Cholesterol: 76 mg

Salad with Orzo and Spinach

INGREDIENTS

3/4 cup chopped fresh parsley
1-1/2 cups uncooked whole wheat orzo pasta
2 green onions, chopped
2 cups grape tomatoes, halved
4 cups fresh baby spinach
14-1/2 ounces reduced-sodium chicken broth
15 ounces each chickpeas, rinsed and drained
DRESSING:
3/4 teaspoon salt
1/4 teaspoon garlic powder
1/4 teaspoon hot pepper sauce
1/4 teaspoon pepper
1/4 cup olive oil
3 tablespoons lemon juice

STEPS

1. In a saucepan, bring broth to a boil. Stir in orzo; return to a boil. Reduce heat; simmer, covered, for 10 minutes.
2. In a bowl, toss spinach and warm orzo, allowing the spinach to wilt slightly. Add chickpeas, tomatoes, green onions, and parsley.
3. Mix in another bowl the olive oil, lemon juice, garlic, hot pepper sauce, salt, and pepper.
4. Sprinkle on the salad. Serve!

NUTRITION FACTS

Per Serving:
Calories: 122
Fat: 5 g
Saturated fat: 1 g
Carbohydrates: 16 g
Fiber: 4 g
Sodium: 259 mg
Cholesterol: 0 mg

Turkey with Asparagus

INGREDIENTS

1/4 cup chicken broth
1 tablespoon lemon juice
1 teaspoon soy sauce
1 garlic clove, minced
1 pound turkey breast tenderloins, cut into 1/2-inch strips
1 pound fresh asparagus, trimmed and cut into 1-1/2-inch pieces
2 tablespoons canola oil, divided
2 teaspoons cornstarch
2 ounces sliced pimientos, drained

STEPS

1. In a bowl, combine the broth, cornstarch, lemon juice, and soy sauce until smooth; set aside. In a skillet wok, turkey, and garlic in 1 tablespoon oil; cook, for 6 minutes, removes, and keep warm.
2. Stir-fry asparagus in remaining oil until crisp-tender. Add pimientos. Stir broth mixture and add to the pan; cook and stir for 1 minute.
3. Return turkey to the pan and toss for 2 minutes.
4. Serve!

NUTRITION FACTS

Per Serving:
Calories: 205
Fat: 9 g
Saturated fat: 1 g
Carbohydrates: 5 g
Fiber: 1 g
Sodium: 204 mg
Cholesterol: 56 mg

Sausage & Onion Spaghetti

INGREDIENTS

3/4 pound Italian turkey sausage links, casings removed
1/2 cup loosely packed fresh basil leaves, thinly sliced
1/2 cup half-and-half cream
1 sweet onion, thinly sliced
1 pint cherry tomatoes, halved
2 teaspoons olive oil
6 ounces uncooked whole wheat spaghetti
Shaved Parmesan cheese for garnish

STEPS

1. Cook spaghetti according to package directions. Meanwhile, in a nonstick skillet over medium heat, cook sausage in oil for 6 minutes. Add onion; cook for 12 minutes longer.
2. Stir in tomatoes and basil; heat through. Add cream; bring to a boil. Drain spaghetti; toss with sausage mixture.
3. Garnish with Parmesan cheese. Serve!

NUTRITION FACTS

Per Serving:
Calories: 334
Fat: 12 g
Saturated fat: 4 g
Carbohydrates: 41 g
Fiber: 6 g
Sodium: 378 mg
Cholesterol: 46 mg

Chicken & Goat Cheese

INGREDIENTS

1/8 teaspoon pepper
1/4 teaspoon salt
1/2 pound boneless skinless chicken breasts, cut into 1-inch pieces
1 cup cut fresh asparagus (1-inch pieces)
1 garlic clove, minced
2 teaspoons olive oil
2 tablespoons herbed fresh goat cheese, crumbled
3 plum tomatoes, chopped
3 tablespoons 2% milk
Hot cooked rice
Additional goat cheese

STEPS

1. Toss chicken with salt and pepper. In a skillet, heat oil over medium heat; saute chicken, for 6 minutes. Remove from pan; keep warm.
2. Add asparagus to skillet; cook and stir over medium heat for 2 minutes. Add garlic; cook and stir for 40 seconds. Stir in tomatoes, milk, and 2 tablespoons cheese; cook, covered, over medium heat, for 3 minutes. Stir in chicken. Serve with rice.
3. Garnish with additional cheese. Serve!

NUTRITION FACTS

Per Serving:
Calories: 251
Fat: 11 g
Saturated Fat: 3 g
Carbohydrates: 8 g
Fiber: 3 g
Sodium: 447 mg
Cholesterol: 74 mg

Cod and Asparagus Bake

INGREDIENTS

1/4 cup grated Romano cheese
1 pound fresh thin asparagus, trimmed
1 pint cherry tomatoes, halved
1-1/2 teaspoons grated lemon zest
2 tablespoons lemon juice
4 cod fillets (4 ounces each)

STEPS

1. Preheat oven to 400 degrees F.
2. Place cod and asparagus in a 15x10x1-in. baking pan brushed with oil. Add tomatoes, cut sides down. Brush fish with lemon juice; sprinkle with lemon zest.
3. Sprinkle fish and vegetables with Romano cheese. Bake, for about 10 minutes.
4. Remove pan from oven; preheat broiler. Broil cod mixture 3-4 in. from heat, for 4 minutes.
5. Serve!

NUTRITION FACTS

Per Serving:
Calories: 141
Fat: 3 g
Saturated fat: 2 g
Carbohydrates: 6 g
Fiber: 2 g
Sodium: 184 mg
Cholesterol: 45 mg

Vegetable & Rice Bowl

INGREDIENTS

1/2 cup sliced baby portobello mush-rooms
1 tablespoon canola oil
1 medium zucchini, julienned
1 cup bean sprouts
1 cup fresh baby spinach
1 tablespoon water
1 tablespoon reduced-sodium soy sauce
1 tablespoon chili garlic sauce
1 teaspoon sesame oil
2 medium carrots, julienned
3 cups hot cooked brown rice
4 large eggs

STEPS

1. In a skillet, heat canola oil over medium heat. Add carrots, zucchini, and mushrooms; cook and stir for 6 minutes. Add the spinach, bean sprouts, water, soy sauce, and chili sauce; cook and stir for about 4 minutes. Remove from heat; keep warm.
2. Place 3 in. of water in a skillet with high sides. Bring to a boil; adjust heat to maintain a gentle simmer. Break cold eggs, 1 at a time, into a bowl; holding bowl close to the surface of the water, slip egg into the water.
3. Cook, uncovered, for 6 minutes. Using a slotted spoon, lift eggs out of water.
4. Serve rice in bowls. Garnish with vegetables. Sprinkle with sesame oil. Top each serving with a poached egg.

NUTRITION FACTS

Per Serving:
Calories: 305
Fat: 11 g
Saturated fat: 2 g
Carbohydrates: 40 g
Fiber: 4 g
Sodium: 364 mg
Cholesterol: 186 mg

Italian-Style Chicken Veggie Packets

INGREDIENTS

1/4 teaspoon pepper
1/2 teaspoon salt
1/2 pound sliced fresh mushrooms
1/2 cup julienned sweet red pepper
1 cup pearl onions
1-1/2 cups fresh baby carrots
3 teaspoons minced fresh thyme
4 boneless skinless chicken breast halves
Lemon wedges

STEPS

1. Preheat oven to 400 degrees F. Flatten chicken breasts to 1/2-in. thickness; place each on a piece of heavy-duty foil.
2. Layer the mushrooms, onions, carrots, and red pepper over chicken; sprinkle with pepper, thyme, and salt.
3. Fold foil around chicken and vegetables and seal tightly. Place on a baking sheet. Bake for 20 minutes.
4. Garnish with lemon wedges. Serve!

NUTRITION FACTS

Per Serving:
Calories: 175
Fat: 3 g
Saturated fat: 1 g
Carbohydrates: 11 g
Fiber: 2 g
Sodium: 100 mg
Cholesterol: 63 mg

Chicken with Celery Puree

INGREDIENTS

2/3 cup unsweetened apple juice
1/4 teaspoon salt
1/2 teaspoon pepper
1 large celery root, peeled and chopped
1 small onion, chopped
2 cups chopped peeled butternut squash
2 garlic cloves, minced
3 teaspoons canola oil, divided
4 boneless skinless chicken breast halves

STEPS

1. Sprinkle chicken with pepper and salt. In a nonstick skillet coated with cooking spray, heat 2 teaspoons oil over medium heat. Brown chicken on both sides. Remove chicken from pan.
2. In the same pan, heat the remaining oil over medium heat. Add celery root, onion, and squash; cook and stir until squash is crisp-tender. Add garlic; cook 1 minute longer.
3. Return chicken to pan; add apple juice. Bring to a boil. Reduce heat; simmer, covered, for 16 minutes.
4. Remove chicken; keep warm. Cool vegetable mixture slightly. Process in a food processor until smooth. Return to pan and heat through.
5. Serve with chicken.

NUTRITION FACTS

Per Serving:
Calories: 328
Fat: 8 g
Saturated fat: 1 g
Carbohydrates: 28 g
Fiber: 5 g
Sodium: 348 mg
Cholesterol: 94 mg

Delicious Spiced Soup

INGREDIENTS

1/2 teaspoon coarsely ground pepper
1/2 teaspoon ground coriander
1 cup dried green split peas
1 teaspoon ground cumin
1 medium onion, chopped
1 celery rib, thinly sliced
2 medium potatoes, chopped
2 medium carrots, halved and thinly sliced
3 garlic cloves, minced
3 bay leaves
4 teaspoons curry powder
28 ounces diced tomatoes, undrained
32 ounces reduced-sodium chicken broth

STEPS

1. In a 4-qt. slow cooker combines the onion, carrots, celery rib, green split peas, cloves, curry, potatoes, bay leaves, cumin, pepper, coriander, and chicken broth. Cook, covered, on low, for about 4 hours.
2. Stir in tomatoes; heat through. Discard bay leaves, and serve!

NUTRITION FACTS

Per Serving:
Calories: 139
Fat: 0 g
Saturated fat: 0 g
Carbohydrates: 27 g
Fiber: 8 g
Sodium: 347 mg
Cholesterol: 0 mg

Chickpea Salad and Mint

INGREDIENTS

1/4 teaspoon pepper
1/4 cup minced fresh mint
1/4 cup olive oil
1/2 teaspoon salt
1/2 cup minced fresh parsley
1 cup fresh peas, thawed
1 cup bulgur
2 cups water
2 tablespoons julienned soft sun-dried tomatoes
2 tablespoons lemon juice
15 ounces chickpeas, rinsed and drained

STEPS

1. In a saucepan, combine bulgur and water; bring to a boil. Reduce heat; simmer, covered, 10 minutes. Stir in fresh peas; cook, covered, for 6 minutes.
2. Transfer to a bowl. Stir the olive oil, lemon juice, fresh peas, bulgur, tomatoes, chickpeas, parsley, fresh mint, salt, and pepper; mix.
3. Serve warm.

NUTRITION FACTS

Per Serving:
Calories: 380
Fat: 16 g
Saturated fat: 2 g
Carbohydrates: 51 g
Fiber: 11 g
Sodium: 450 mg
Cholesterol: 0 mg

CPSIA information can be obtained
at www.ICGtesting.com
Printed in the USA
BVHW051949250521
608097BV00003B/610